Neuroscience
PreTest®
Self-Assessment
and Review

NOTICE

Medicine is an ever-changing science. As new research and clinical experience broaden our knowledge, changes in treatment and drug therapy are required. The authors, editor, and publisher of this work have checked with sources believed to be reliable in their efforts to provide information that is complete and generally in accord with the standards accepted at the time of publication. However, in view of the possibility of human error or changes in medical sciences, neither the editors nor the publisher nor any other party who has been involved in the preparation or publication of this work warrants that the information contained herein is in every respect accurate or complete, and they are not responsible for any errors or omissions or for the results obtained from use of such information. Readers are encouraged to confirm the information contained herein with other sources. For example and in particular, readers are advised to check the product information sheet included in the package of each drug they plan to administer to be certain that the information contained in this book is accurate and that changes have not been made in the recommended dose or in the contraindications for administration. This recommendation is of particular importance in connection with new or infrequently used drugs.

Neuroscience

PreTest®
Self-Assessment
and Review

Allan Siegel, Ph.D.
Department of Neuroscience
New Jersey Medical School
Newark, New Jersey

McGraw-Hill, Inc.
Health Professions Division/PreTest® Series

New York   St. Louis   San Francisco   Auckland
Bogotá   Caracas   Lisbon   London   Madrid
Mexico   Milan   Montreal   New Delhi   Paris
San Juan   Singapore   Sydney   Tokyo   Toronto

Neuroscience: PreTest® Self-Assessment and Review

2 3 4 5 6 7 8 9 0 DOCDOC 9 8 7 6 5 4 3

ISBN 0-07-051995-1

The editors were Gail Gavert and John R. Thornborough.
The production supervisors were
Clara B. Stanley and Gyl Favours
R.R. Donnelley & Sons was printer and binder.
This book was set in Times Roman by ILOC, Inc.

Library of Congress Cataloging-in-Publication Data

Siegel, Allan.
    Neuroscience : PreTest self assessment and review / Allan Siegel .
-- 1st ed.
      p. cm. -- (Clinical sciences series)
    Includes bibliographical references.
    ISBN 0-07-051995-1 :
    1. Neurophysiology--Examinations, questions, etc. I. Title.
II. Series.
    [DNLM: 1. Nervous System--anatomy & histology--examination
questions. 2. Nervous System--physiology--examination questions.
WL 18 S571n]
OP356.S49 1992
612.8--dc20
DNLM/DLC
for Library of Congress   92-3048
                                            CIP

DEDICATION

To my wife Carla,

whose patience, support, and understanding made this book possible

Contents

Preface

The study of the neurosciences has undergone remarkable growth over the past two decades. To a large extent, such advancements have been made possible through the development of new methodologies; especially in the fields of neuropharmacology, molecular biology, and neuroanatomy. Neuroscience courses presented in medical schools and related schools of health professions generally are unable to cover all of the material that has evolved in recent years. For this reason, *Neuroscience: PreTest® Self-Assessment and Review* was written for medical students preparing for national boards as well as for undergraduate students in the health professions.

The subject matter of this book is mainly the classical topics of anatomy and physiology of the nervous system. Also, an attempt was made to encompass the subjects of molecular and biophysical properties of membranes, neuropharmacology, and higher functions of the nervous system. Moreover, clinical correlations for each part of the central nervous system, often utilizing MRI and CT scans, are presented. While it is virtually impossible to cover all aspects of the neurosciences, the objective of this book was to include its most significant components as we currently understand them.

The author wishes to express his gratitude to Majid B. Shaikh, Ph.D., for his modifications of the line drawings and to Leo Wolansky, M.D. and Alan Zimmer, M.D. for providing the MRI's and CT scans.

Introduction

Neuroscience: *PreTest® Self-Assessment and Review* has been designed to provide medical students, as well as physicians, with a comprehensive and convenient instrument for self- assessment and review within the field of neuroscience. The over 500 questions provided have been designed to parallel the format and degree of difficulty of the questions contained in Step 1 of the United States Medical Licensing Examination (USMLE) and the Foreign Medical Graduate Examination in the Medical Sciences (FMGEMS).

Each question in the book is accompanied by an answer, a paragraph explanation, and a specific page reference to a textbook. A bibliography listing the sources used in the book follows the last chapter. Perhaps the most effective way to use this book is to allow yourself one minute to answer each question in a given chapter; as you proceed, indicate your answer beside each question. By following this suggestion, you will be approximating the time limits imposed by the board examinations previously mentioned.

When you finish answering the questions in a chapter, you should then spend as much time as you need verifying your answers and carefully reading the explanations. Although you should pay special attention to the explanations for the questions you answered incorrectly, you should read *every* explanation. The author of this book has designed the explanations to reinforce and supplement the information tested by the questions. If, after reading the explanations for a given chapter, you feel you need still more information about the material covered, you should consult and study the references indicated.

Neuroscience
PreTest®
Self-Assessment
and Review

Brain Gross Anatomy

DIRECTIONS: Each group of questions below consists of lettered headings followed by a set of numbered items. For each numbered item select the **one** lettered point on the figure with which it is **most** closely associated. Each lettered item may be used **once, more than once, or not at all**.

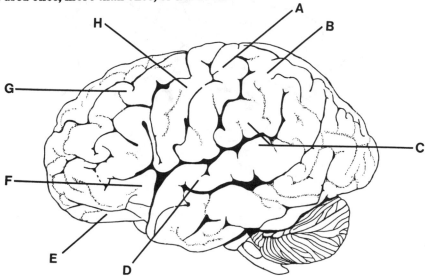

(Adapted from DeArmond et al., Fig. 10-2; with permission.)

Questions 1-9   Refer to the figure above.

1. Cells in this region give rise to fibers which supply the cervical cord.

2. This region receives somatosensory inputs from the lower limb.

3. A lesion of this region will likely result in "receptive" aphasia.

4. Destruction of the cells in this region frequently results in loss of ability to formulate a plan for the execution of a complex act.

5. A lesion at this site is often characterized by a "flattening" of emotional reactions, carelessness in personal habits, and a lack of interest in future events.

6. "Motor" speech area.

7. Electrical stimulation of this region causes conjugate deviation of the eyes.

8. Histological study has shown this region is almost devoid of pyramidal cells.

9. This region receives major input from ventrolateral nucleus of the thalamus.

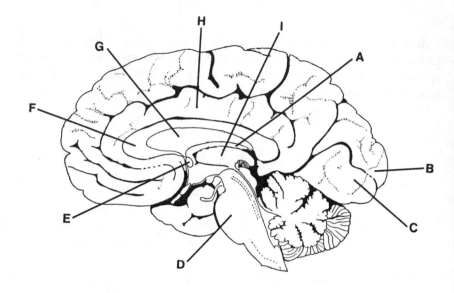

(Adapted from DeArmond et al., Fig. 4; with permission.)

Questions 10-17   Refer to the figure above.

10. A commissure of the brain conveying olfactory information.

11. This structure forms the medial wall of the lateral ventricle.

12. This cortical structure is considered part of the limbic lobe and receives a significant input from the anteroventral thalamic nucleus.

13. Loss of cells in this region results in loss of vision in the lower visual field.

14. This structure projects axons to the mammillary bodies and anterior thalamic complex.

15. This structure is an important relay for cortical inputs to the cerebellum.

16. A lesion of the temporal lobe will disrupt primary sensory inputs to this region.

17. The transfer of information from the dominant to the nondominant hemisphere utilizes this fiber system.

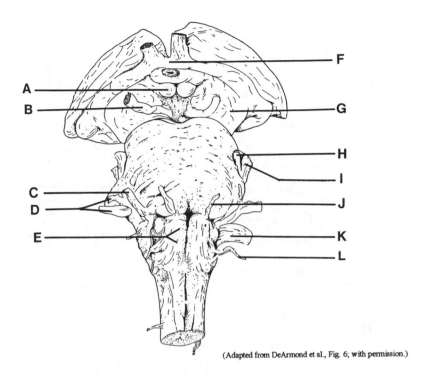

(Adapted from DeArmond et al., Fig. 6; with permission.)

Questions 18-28   Refer to the figure above.

18. This fiber bundle contains axons from neurons in the nucleus ambiguus.

19. This structure controls muscles of mastication.

20. The axons from neurons in this structure project to the anteroventral thalamic nucleus.

21. This nerve controls the muscles of facial expression.

22. The fibers in this region may terminate in the midbrain, pons, medulla, or spinal cord.

23. These fibers carry pain and temperature sensation from the face.

24. A lesion at this site will cause ipsilateral loss of medial gaze.

25. Damage to these fibers will cause ipsilateral loss of lateral gaze.

26. A tumor at this site can result in a bitemporal hemianopsia.

27. These are first-order sensory neurons arising from the semicircular canals.

28. Damage to these fibers results in a deviation of the tongue to the side of the lesion.

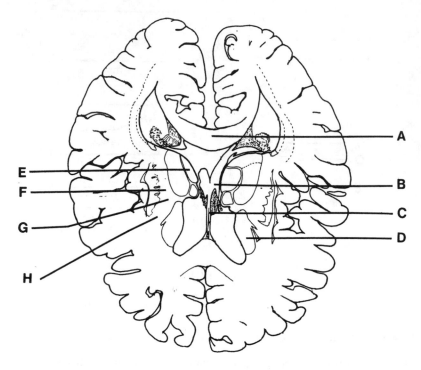

(Adapted from DeArmond et al., Fig. 15; with permission.)

Questions 29-35   Refer to the figure above.

29. Contains fibers that arise from the leg region of the precentral gyrus.

30. The fibers situated in this region terminate in the pons.

31. A lesion at this site could produce a pseudobulbar palsy.

32. The fibers in this region arise from the hippocampal formation.

33. This structure receives major inputs from the compact division of the substantia nigra and the cerebral cortex.

34. This region makes reciprocal connections with the frontal lobe.

35. The fibers in this region are considered upper motor neurons for the regulation of the muscles of the face.

DIRECTIONS: Each question below contains five suggested responses. Select the one best response to each question.

36. All of the following structures contribute to the walls of the lateral ventricle EXCEPT:

(A) caudate nucleus

(B) corpus callosum

(C) habenula nucleus

(D) fornix

(E) septum pellucidum

37. All of the following about cerebrospinal fluid (CSF) are true EXCEPT:

(A) The general direction of flow of CSF through the brain may be described as: formed in the fourth ventricle; flows through the cerebral aqueduct, third ventricle, and lateral ventricles; and exits primarily through the arachnoid granulations

(B) The formation of CSF takes places in the choroid plexus

(C) CSF is absorbed through arachnoid granulations

(D) The ultimate composition of the CSF is dependent to a considerable extent upon the blood-brain barrier

(E) CSF flows into the subarachnoid spaces at the level of the fourth ventricle through several apertures known as the "foramen of Magendie" and "foramina of Luschka"

38. All of the following about hydrocephalus are true EXCEPT:

(A) it may result from oversecretion of cerebrospinal fluid (CSF)

(B) it may result from a failure of absorption of CSF

(C) it may result from tumor formation within the intraventricular foramen

(D) it may result from tumor formation in the region of the cerebral aqueduct

(E) hydrocephalus can result in brain damage in the adult but not in the infant, because the infant's cranial sutures have not fused

39. All of the following about circumventricular organs are true EXCEPT:

(A) they are specialized tissue situated proximal to the ventricular system

(B) they are not limited only to the brainstem but, in fact, are located at various levels of the central nervous system

(C) one of the circumventricular organs, the organum vasculosum, plays an important role in endocrine regulation by the hypothalamus

(D) the area postrema plays a role in emetic functions

(E) although circumventricular organs are highly vascular, they are generally protected by a well-developed blood-brain barrier system

40. All of the following are components of or functionally related to the basal ganglia EXCEPT:

(A) caudate nucleus

(B) red nucleus

(C) substantia nigra

(D) putamen

(E) subthalamic nucleus

41. All of the following are properties of the choroid plexus EXCEPT:

(A) under hydrostatic pressure, it produces CSF

(B) it consists of a single layer of cuboidal epithelial tissue

(C) it contains a barrier to passive exchange of proteins which is formed by tight junctions surrounding apical regions of the epithelial cells

(D) it contributes to the mechanism governing peptide regulation of the pituitary by the hypothalamus

(E) an active Na^+/K^+ pump is present which accounts for the relatively higher concentration of Na^+ in choroidal secretions

42. The walls that form the cisterns encasing the brain include:

(A) ependyma and nerve cells

(B) dura mater and ependyma

(C) pia mater and arachnoid

(D) arachnoid and ependyma

(E) pia mater, arachnoid, and dura mater

43. Which of the following statements about the blood-brain barrier is correct?

(A) It has well-developed capillary pores that allow for selective diffusion of substances.

(B) It is selectively permeable to certain compounds such as biogenic amines.

(C) It is found within all structures enclosed by the meninges, including the pineal gland.

(D) Tight junctions associated with the blood-brain barrier are formed exclusively by neuronal or glial processes.

(E) The blood-brain barrier is generally limited to highly vascular regions of the brain such as those present at the level of the ventromedial hypothalamus.

Brain Gross Anatomy

Answers

1-9. The answers are: 1-H, 2-A, 3-C, 4-B, 5-E, 6-F, 7-G, 8-A, 9-H. (Carpenter and Sutin, 8th Ed., pp. 653, 656-658, 660, 684-687, 689-693, 701-705) This figure is a lateral view of the cerebral cortex. Cells in the "arm" area of the primary motor cortex (H) project their axons to the cervical level of the spinal cord. This area receives major input from the ventrolateral nucleus of the thalamus. The "leg" region of the primary somatosensory cortex (A) lies immediately caudal to the central sulcus, is almost devoid of pyramidal cells, and is referred to as a "granulous" cortex. The cells situated in the region of the dorsal border of the superior temporal gyrus and adjoining area of the inferior parietal lobule (Wernicke's area) (C) regulate speech mechanisms. Lesions of this region frequently result in a form of speech deficit called "receptive aphasia." The posterior parietal lobule (B) is important because it sends integrated signals to the premotor region. A lesion in the posterior parietal lobule results in an inability to formulate and execute a complex motor act. The orbital frontal cortex (E) lies in a position inferior and rostral to Broca's motor speech area. This region governs general intellectual functions and emotional behavior. An additional region of the cortex governing speech — the "motor speech area" (Broca's area) (F) — is situated in the inferior aspect of the frontal lobe immediately rostral and slightly ventral to the precentral gyrus. The caudal aspect of the middle frontal gyrus (G) contains cells that, when activated, produce conjugate deviation of the eyes.

10-17. The answers are: 10-E, 11-G, 12-H, 13-B, 14-A, 15-D, 16-C, 17-F. (Carpenter and Sutin, 8th Ed., pp. 28-39, 51-60, 461-463, 505-507, 543-544, 560-563, 699-700) This figure is a mid-sagittal section of the brain. A major portion of the anterior commissure (E) contains fibers which arise from the olfactory bulb and decussate to the contralateral olfactory bulb. The septum pellucidum (G) forms the medial wall of the lateral ventricle, which in fact, separates the lateral ventricle on one side from that on the opposite side. The cingulate gyrus (H) is a prominent structure on the medial aspect of the cerebral cortex and comprises a major component of the limbic lobe. It receives a significant input from the antero-ventral thalamic nucleus. The upper bank of the calcarine fissure (B) receives fibers from the lateral geniculate nucleus and comprises that aspect of the primary visual cortex associated with the lower visual fields. The fibers from the lateral geniculate

8 Neuroscience

nucleus, which supply the lower bank of the calcarine fissure (C) and are associated with upper visual fields, traverse portions of the temporal lobe. For this reason, lesions of the temporal lobe can cause an upper visual field deficit. Fibers of the fornix (A) arise from the subicular cortex and adjoining portions of hippocampal formation and are distributed to the anterior thalamic complex, mammillary bodies, and septal area. The basilar portion of the pons (D) constitutes the ventral half of this region of the brainstem and contains neurons receiving afferents from wide regions of the neocortex. The axons of these pontine neurons project to the cerebellum. The basilar aspect of the pons serves as an important relay nucleus for inputs from the cerebral cortex to the cerebellum. Communication between the two cerebral hemispheres is mediated via fibers of the corpus callosum (F).

18-28. The answers are: 18-K, 19-H, 20-A, 21-C, 22-G, 23-I, 24-B, 25-J, 26-F, 27-D, 28-L. (Carpenter and Sutin, 8th Ed., pp.34-51, 283-284, 315-318) This figure is a ventral view of the brainstem. Fibers that arise from the nucleus ambiguus exit the brain on the lateral side of the medulla as part of the vagus nerve (K) and innervate the muscles of the pharynx and larynx as special visceral efferents. The motor root of the trigeminal nerve exits the brain laterally at the mid-pontine level. The motor root (H), which lies medial to the sensory root, innervates the muscles of mastication. The mammillary bodies (A), which lie on the ventral surface of the brain at the caudal aspect of the hypothalamus, project many of their axons to the anteroventral thalamic nucleus as the mammillothalamic tract. The facial nerve (C) exits the brain at the level of the ventrolateral aspect of the caudal pons and its special visceral efferent component innervates the muscles of facial expression. The cerebral peduncle (G) is situated in the ventrolateral aspect of the midbrain and contains fibers of cortical origin that project to all levels of the neuraxis of the brainstem and spinal cord. First-order sensory fibers from the face (I), which include the modalities of pain and temperature, enter the brain laterally at the level of the middle of the pons as the sensory root of the trigeminal nerve. The oculomotor nerve (B) exits the brain at the level of the ventromedial aspect of the midbrain and some of the fibers of the general somatic efferent component of this nerve innervate the medial rectus muscle. Damage to this component causes a loss of medial gaze. The abducent nerve (J) exits the brain from a ventromedial position at the level of the medulla-pontine border and its fibers innervate the lateral rectus muscle. Damage to this nerve produces a loss of lateral gaze. The optic chiasm (F) contains crossing fibers from the retina that are associated with the temporal (i.e., lateral) visual fields. Therefore, damage to the optic chiasm will produce a bitemporal hemianopsia. First-order neurons from the semicircular canals (D) form the vestibular component of cranial nerve VIII, entering the brain laterally at the level of the upper medulla. The hypoglossal nerve (L) exits the brain at the level of the middle of the medulla between the pyramid and the olive. These fibers innervate muscles which move the tongue toward the opposite side. Thus, a lesion of this nerve will result in a deviation of the tongue to the side of the lesion because of the unopposed action of the intact contralateral hypoglossal nerve.

29-35. The answers are: 29-F, 30-H, 31-G, 32-B, 33-D, 34-E, 35-G. (Carpenter and Sutin, 8th Ed., pp. 354, 508-509, 537-538, 602-603, 630-631) This figure is a horizontal view of the brain at the level of the head of the caudate nucleus and the internal capsule. The posterior limb of the internal capsule(F) contains fibers which arise from the leg region of cerebral cortex and project to lumbar levels of spinal cord, thus serving as upper motor neurons for the elicitation of voluntary movement of the contralateral leg. Fibers in the anterior limb of the internal capsule(H) project in large numbers to deep pontine nuclei and represent first order neurons in a pathway linking the cerebral cortex with the cerebellum. Pseudobulbar palsy is characterized in part by a weakness of the muscles controlling swallowing, chewing, breathing, and speaking and results from a lesion of the upper motor neurons associated with the head region of the cortex which pass through the genu of the internal capsule (G) en route to brainstem cranial nerve nuclei upon which they synapse. The descending column of the fornix (B), situated along the midline of the brain, contains fibers which arise from the hippocampal formation. The head of the caudate nucleus (D) is part of an important element of the motor systems called the basal ganglia. It receives significant inputs from other regions associated with motor functions such as the cerebral cortex and the dopamine containing region of the substantia nigra (i.e., pars compacta). The mediodorsal thalamic nucleus (E) receives significant inputs from the prefrontal cortex and, in turn, projects its axons in large quantities back to that region of the cortex. Fibers contained in the genu of the internal capsule(G) serve as upper motor neurons for motor functions associated with cranial nerve motor nuclei, including those involving the facial muscles.

36. The answer is C. (Carpenter and Sutin, 8th Ed., pp. 41-45) The roof of the lateral ventricle is formed by the corpus callosum, its lateral wall by the caudate nucleus, its medial wall by the fornix and septum pellucidum. The habenula nucleus is situated below the fornix and thus is not contiguous to the lateral ventricle.

37. The answer is A. (Kandel, 3rd Ed., pp. 1050-1055; Carpenter and Sutin, 8th Ed., pp. 41-48) The general flow of CSF is from the lateral ventricle, where most of the CSF is produced from the choroid plexus, down through the third ventricle, cerebral aqueduct, and fourth ventricle where it exits the brain through the foramina of Luschka and foramen of Magendie into the subarachnoid space. CSF is also absorbed into the superior sagittal sinus and other venous structures through arachnoid granulations which appear as herniations of the arachnoid membrane. Since CSF and extracellular fluids of the brain are in equilibrium, changes in the blood-brain barrier will alter this equilibrium. Such effects become apparent in certain disease states. For example, in the case of multiple sclerosis, gamma globulin content of the CSF increases to more than 13% of total protein and can be used as a diagnostic indicator.

38. The answer is E. (Kandel, 3rd Ed., pp. 1059-1060; Carpenter and Sutin, 8th Ed., p. 18) It is theoretically possible for hydrocephalus to result from the oversecretion of CSF or failure of absorption of CSF. Oversecretion of CSF does, in fact, occasionally occur in such circumstances where tumor formation involves the choroid plexus. Impaired absorption may result from a number of conditions, including a mechanical impairment of the subarachnoid granulations. The most common form of hydrocephalus results from blockade of CSF pathways — often as the result of tumors or congenital malformations. In infants, hydrocephalus can lead to very serious neurological impairment of the newly formed (and perhaps still developing) neural tissue. Additionally, hydrocephalus may cause a change in the shape of the cranium which has not completely fused in infants.

39. The answer is E. (Carpenter and Sutin, 8th Ed., pp. 23-24) Circumventricular organs are specialized tissue generally situated along the midline of the ventricular system at different levels along the neuraxis of the brain. The functions of several of these structures have been studied in detail. For example, it is now known that the organum vasculosum serves as a possible route by which certain hormones are regulated by the hypothalamus. In particular, luteinizing hormone releasing hormone and somatostatin apparently utilize this structure as a vascular outlet by which their influence upon the pituitary is ultimately achieved. The area postrema has been shown to play an important role in the regulation of emetic functions. The unusual feature of circumventricular organs is they lack a blood-brain barrier.

40. The answer is B. (Carpenter and Sutin, 8th Ed., pp. 51-56, 579-586, 591-593) The caudate nucleus and the putamen are considered to be major receiving areas of information that enters the basal ganglia. The substantia nigra and subthalamic nucleus have important reciprocal connections with parts of the basal ganglia. By virtue of such connections, these structures play important regulatory roles in the motor functions associated with the basal ganglia. While the red nucleus is an important structure with respect to motor functions, its actions appear to be independent of those of the basal ganglia.

41. The answer is D. (Carpenter and Sutin, 8th Ed., pp. 14-20) The choroid plexus, which consists of a single layer of cuboidal epithelial cells, produces cerebrospinal fluid under hydrostatic pressure. The barrier to passive transport or exchange of proteins and certain other substances such as hydrophilic solutes is formed by the tight junctions connecting apical regions of these epithelial cells. The fact that choroidal secretions contain relatively higher Na^+ and relatively lower K^+ is accounted for by an active sodium-potassium pump. Peptide regulation of pituitary functions is unrelated to the general functions of the choroid plexus.

42. The answer is C. (Carpenter and Sutin, 8th Ed., pp. 6-16) The meninges of the brain include pia mater, arachnoid, and dura mater. Pia mater and arachnoid are situated closest to the brain and dura mater is in an external position. Normally, the space between the pia and arachnoid is called subarachnoid space and is filled with cerebrospinal fluid. Surrounding the brain, the subarachnoid space shows local variations. At places where bulges are present, they are referred to as cisterns.

43. The answer is B. (Carpenter and Sutin, 8th Ed., pp. 18-23; Kandel, 3rd Ed., pp. 1054-1056) The blood-brain barrier is selectively permeable to certain types of substances such as biogenic amines and not to others. The barrier is formed by tight junctions consisting of capillary endothelial cells that are frequently in contact with the glial end-feet of astrocytes. The barrier does not contain well-developed capillary pores. It is not found within circumventricular organs such as the subfornical organ and the pineal gland but is applied to all other brain tissues.

Development

DIRECTIONS: Each group of questions below consists of lettered headings followed by a set of numbered items. For each numbered item select the **one** lettered heading with which it is **most** closely associated. Each lettered item may be used **once, more than once, or not at all**.

Questions 44-54

(A) alar plate
(B) basal plate
(C) floor plate
(D) roof plate
(E) neural crest cells
(F) mesencephalon
(G) rhombic lips
(H) Rathke's pouch
(I) telencephalon
(J) sulcus limitans
(K) isocortex

44. alpha motor neurons

45. proper sensory nucleus

46. dorsal root ganglia

47. spinal nucleus (cranial nerve V)

48. hypoglossal nucleus (cranial nerve XII)

49. cerebellum

50. sympathetic ganglia

51. choroid plexus

52. chromaffin cells of adrenal medulla

53. amygdala

54. anterior pituitary

Development

Answers

44-54. The answers are: 44-B, 45-A, 46-E, 47-A, 48-B, 49-A or H, 50-E, 51-D, 52-E, 53-I, 54-H. (Carpenter and Sutin, 8th Ed., pp. 64-67, 69-75,81) Structures associated with motor functions such as alpha motor neurons and the hypoglossal nucleus are derived from the basal plate (B). Structures associated with sensory functions such as the proper sensory nucleus of the dorsal horn of the spinal cord and spinal nucleus of the trigeminal nerve are derived from the alar plate(A). A number of structures such as the dorsal root ganglia, sympathetic ganglia, and chromaffin cells of the adrenal medulla are derived from neural crest cells (E). The cerebellum is formed from the dorsolateral aspects of the alar plates (A) which bend medially and posteriorly to form the rhombic lips (G). The choroid plexus of the third and lateral ventricles, which is attached to the roof of these ventricles, is derived from the roof plate (D) of the diencephalon. The amygdala is derived from that part of the forebrain called the telencephalon (I). The anterior lobe of the pituitary is formed as an inpocket derivative of the ectodermal stomodeum called Rathke's pouch (H).

The Neuron

DIRECTIONS: Each group of questions below consists of lettered headings followed by a set of numbered items. For each numbered item select the **one** lettered heading with which it is **most** closely associated. Each lettered item may be used **once, more than once, or not at all**.

55-60. The following questions relate to methods utilized for the anatomical or functional tracing of neurons within the nervous system.

(A) retrograde labeling of cell bodies

(B) metabolic mapping of CNS pathways

(C) anterograde labeling of degenerating axons

(D) labels cell bodies and processes of neurons and glia

(E) labels motor nerve endings

(F) visualization of demyelination

55. Fink-Heimer method

56. horseradish peroxidase (HRP) histochemistry

57. MR imaging

58. 2-deoxyglucose autoradiography

59. gold chloride method

60. Golgi method

DIRECTIONS: Each question below contains five suggested responses. Select the one best response to each question.

61. All of the following events occur during the process of retrograde degeneration EXCEPT:

(A) a displacement of the nucleus toward the periphery of the cell

(B) initially, the cell body begins swelling

(C) a proliferation of Nissl granules

(D) degeneration of processes along the axon distal to the lesion

(E) there is an initial accumulation of mitochondria in the axoplasm at the nodes of Ranvier

62. All of the following statements concerning myelin are true EXCEPT:

(A) in the peripheral nervous system, myelin is formed from Schwann cells

(B) the plasmalemma of the Schwann cell surrounds an axon and spirals around the axon in concentric layers

(C) the spaces between Schwann cells will become nodes of Ranvier

(D) the same group of proteins are found in myelin of both the central and peripheral nervous systems

(E) in oligodendrocytes the genes that encode myelin are "turned on" by the presence of axons

63. All of the following statements about nerve cells are true EXCEPT:

(A) Messenger RNA molecules for cytosolic proteins emerge from the nuclear pores and become associated with ribosomes to form free polysomes in the cytoplasm.

(B) Cytosolic proteins show little modification or processing following their translation.

(C) Secretory proteins also undergo little or no modification or processing after translation.

(D) Nuclear and mitochondrial proteins that are encoded by the cell's nucleus are targeted to their proper organelle by a process called posttranslational importation.

(E) More than one copy of the same peptide as well as different peptides may be cut from the same precursor molecule.

64. The trigger zone that integrates incoming signals from other cells and initiates the signal that the neuron sends to another neuron or muscle cell corresponds to:

(A) cell body

(B) dendritic trunk

(C) dendritic spines

(D) axon hillock and initial segment

(E) axon trunk

65. All of the following statements concerning axoplasmic transport are correct EXCEPT:

(A) Evidence suggests it is not likely that microtubules are involved in the retrograde transport of particles.

(B) There exists a slow transport system that involves the movement of soluble enzymes and proteins.

(C) There exists a fast transport system which involves the movement of newly synthesized membranous organelles within the axon.

(D) A considerable percentage of the material transported consists of synaptic vesicles or their precursors destined for the axon terminals.

(E) Fast axoplasmic transport has been shown to have bidirectional movement (in both anterograde and retrograde directions).

66. All of the following are likely to be involved in the gating of channels EXCEPT:

(A) binding of a ligand to its receptor

(B) continuous exposure to high concentration of a given ligand

(C) protein phosphorylation and dephosphorylation

(D) mechanical force that stretches the membrane

(E) conformational changes in the channel proteins

67. All of the following statements concerning ion channels are correct EXCEPT:

(A) The ion flux through ion channels is generally regarded as a highly active process that requires the expenditure of metabolic energy.

(B) Most cation channels are selective in that they are permeable to a single type of ion.

(C) Ion flow is normally characterized by the nature of the voltage-dependence of the channel's conductance.

(D) The electrochemical driving force is determined by the electrical potential difference and the chemical concentration gradient of the ions across the membrane.

(E) Ionic flow through a single channel saturates at higher concentrations of that ion.

68. Which of the following statements concerning the membrane time constant is correct:

(A) The time constant is a function of the membrane's resistance and capacitance.

(B) The time constant is unrelated to the membrane capacitance.

(C) The time course of the rising phase of a synaptic potential is specifically dependent upon the time constant for that cell.

(D) The falling phase of a synaptic potential is dependent upon active and passive membrane properties.

(E) The integration of synaptic potentials is unrelated to the length of the time constant.

69. All of the following statements concerning the membrane potential are true EXCEPT:

(A) The resting membrane potential is directly proportional to separation of charge across the membrane.

(B) A membrane is depolarized when the separation of charge across the membrane is reduced.

(C) As inside of the cell is made more negative with respect to outside, the cell becomes depolarized.

(D) In a cell in which its membrane possesses only K^+ channels, the membrane potential will approach the K^+ equilibrium potential.

(E) Passive fluxes of Na^+ and K^+ are balanced by an active pump that derives energy from enzymatic hydrolysis of ATP.

70. All of the following statements concerning length constants are true EXCEPT:

(A) Length constant is the distance along a dendrite where the change in membrane potential produced by a current decays to approximately 1/3 of its original value.

(B) Length constant increases as the membrane resistance decreases.

(C) Length constant decreases as the axial resistance increases.

(D) Length constant is greater in myelinated than in unmyelinated fibers.

(E) As the length constant increases in a postsynaptic neuron, the efficiency of electrotonic conduction of synaptic potentials (at that synapse) also increases.

71. Which of the following statements concerning sodium channels is true:

(A) They are opened when the membrane is hyperpolarized.

(B) They display a high conductance in the resting membrane.

(C) They open rapidly following depolarization of the membrane.

(D) They are rapidly inactivated by tetraethylammonium.

(E) They are rapidly activated by tetrodotoxin.

72. The equilibrium potential for potassium, as determined by the Nernst Equation, differs from the resting potential of the neuron because:

(A) an active sodium-potassium pump makes an important contribution to the regulation of the resting potential

(B) the membrane is permeable to ions other than potassium

(C) the Nernst Equation basically considers only the relative distribution of potassium ions across the membrane

(D) the resting potential is basically dependent upon the concentration of sodium but not potassium ions across the membrane

(E) the Nernst Equation fails to account for local changes in temperature that influence the resting membrane potential

Questions 73-76 Kuffler studied the electrophysiology of glial cells, using the optic nerve and its surrounding glial sheath. He found that the mean value of the resting potential of these cells, as recorded by intracellular microelectrodes, was –89.6 mV. The potassium concentration in the bathing solution was 3 mEq/L. Assume that RT/F = 61.

73. Assuming that the resting potential is equivalent to the potassium equilibrium potential, calculate the approximate intracellular potassium concentration (in mEq/L):

(A) 11

(B) 33

(C) 88

(D) 140

(E) 155

74. What would be the concentration of potassium (mEq/L) in the bathing fluid in order to depolarize the membrane potential to zero?

(A) 11

(B) 33

(C) 88

(D) 140

(E) 155

75. Stimulation of the optic nerve with a volley of impulses caused a slow and long-lasting depolarization of the associated glial cells. The mean value of the depolarization was 12.1 mV. If this depolarization was due solely to an increase in potassium ion concentration in the intracellular clefts, calculate the change in the concentration of potassium in the extracellular environment (in mEq/L).

(A) 1.79

(B) 36.30

(C) 137.00

(D) 140.50

(E) 5.35×10^{-6}

76. A probable explanation for the depolarization of glial cells following stimulation of nerve fibers is that:

(A) it is a result of a delayed increase in potassium conductance

(B) it is a result of early sodium influx

(C) it is a result of a large efflux of sodium ions

(D) it is the product of temporal summation that results in a long-lasting depolarization

(E) it is a result of an influx of chloride ions

77. Which of the following statements concerning ligand-gating of neuronal membrane channels is true :

(A) The normal triggering mechanism for gating involves nonspecific binding by large classes of molecules.

(B) Channels are opened when a given molecule selectively binds with the gating molecule.

(C) Ligand-gating is triggered by changes in the electrical potential across the membrane.

(D) The channels are constructed of a mixture of proteins and lipids.

(E) The "gating" molecule shows no conformational change during the gating process.

78. After the occurrence of an action potential, there is a repolarization of the membrane. The principal explanation for this event is:

(A) that potassium channels have been opened

(B) that sodium channels have been opened

(C) that the membrane becomes impermeable to all ions

(D) that potassium channels have been inactivated

(E) that there has been a sudden influx of calcium

79. During an *in vitro* experiment, the membrane potential of a nerve cell is hyperpolarized to –120 mV. At that time, a transmitter, known to be inhibitory in function, is applied to the preparation and results in a depolarization of the membrane. The most likely reason for this occurrence is that:

(A) inhibitory transmitters normally depolarize the postsynaptic membrane

(B) the normal response of the postsynaptic membrane to any transmitter is depolarization

(C) calcium channels become activated

(D) sodium channels become inactivated

(E) the inhibitory transmitter activates ligand-gated potassium channels

The Neuron

Answers

55-60. The answers are: 55-C, 56-A, 57-F, 58-B, 59-E, 60-D. (Carpenter and Sutin, 8th Ed., pp. 87-92) The Fink-Heimer technique was used for a number of years as the method of choice for the anterograde tracing of degenerating axons from the site where the lesion was placed to the terminal endings of the damaged axons (C). In this method, the selective silver impregnation of degenerating axons permits visualization of the axons in question. With HRP histochemistry, the glycoprotein enzyme, horseradish peroxidase, is injected into the region of the terminal endings of the neuronal pathway under examination and is incorporated into the axons through a process of micropinocytosis. HRP is then retrogradely transported back to the cell bodies of origin of that pathway (A) where it is then degraded. By reacting the tissue with an appropriate substrate, the labeled cells can be visualized under light microscopy. The Golgi silver method has been widely used to visualize individual neurons and glia (D). It fills the neuron (or glial cell) with a black deposit that extends to the dendrites and axon, thus enabling the observer to clearly characterize the morphological properties of these neurons. 2-deoxyglucose (2DG) autoradiography is used to metabolically map (B) pathways and structures that are functionally active as a result of sensory, chemical, or electrical stimulation of nervous tissue. Local variations in energy metabolism can be visualized because the glucose analog, ^{14}C-2- deoxyglucose (2DG), is phosphorylated to 2DG-6-phosphate where it is not further metabolized and is retained in the neuron. The rate of incorporation into neurons is related to the rate of glucose utilization which is, itself, a function of energy metabolism. The gold chloride method is a histochemical procedure that can be used for visualizing motor nerve endings in skeletal muscle (E). In this method, tissues are placed into a silver-protein solution in which the silver is reduced. When the tissue is passed through a solution of gold chloride, the gold replaces the silver particles in the nerve tissue of that section of tissue. Non-neural gold particles are removed by treatment with oxalic acid. Nerve cells and their processes can be clearly identified using this method. MR imaging permits the visualization of the degenerative process that results in demyelination of axons (F).

61. The answer is C. (Carpenter and Sutin, 8th Ed., pp. 126-128) A number of changes occur in the neuron during the process of retrograde degeneration. The cell body initially shows some swelling and becomes distended. At the beginning of the degenerative process, there is an accumulation of mitochondria in the axoplasm at the nodes of Ranvier. The nucleus is then displaced toward the periphery of the cell. The Nissl granules break down, first in the center of the cell, and later, the breakdown spreads outward. In addition, the axonal process distal to the site of the lesion will undergo degeneration. It should be noted that retrograde degeneration procedures were used experimentally prior to the advent of histochemical methods for identifying cell bodies of origin of given pathways in the CNS.

62. The answer is E. (Kandel, 3rd Ed., pp. 38-44) In the peripheral nervous system, Schwann cells are responsible for producing myelin, while in the CNS, this function is carried out by oligodendrocytes. The myelin present along nerve fibers in both the peripheral and central nervous systems contains the same group of proteins — referred to as "myelin basic protein." Myelin is formed when the plasmalemma of the Schwann cell elongates and spirals around the axon in concentric layers. The nodes of Ranvier are spaces between Schwann cells where the axon is unsheathed. One major difference between Schwann cells and oligodendrocytes is that Schwann cell genes that encode myelin are "turned on" by other Schwann cells, while the genes in oligodendrocytes that encode myelin depend upon the presence of astrocytes rather than other axons.

63. The answer is C. (Kandel, 3rd Ed., pp. 49-56) Cytosolic proteins are the most extensive type of protein in the cell and include those that make up the cytoskeleton and enzymes that catalyze the different metabolic reactions of the cell. Messenger RNAs for these proteins pass through nuclear pores, become associated with ribosomes, and ultimately form free polysomes in the cytoplasm of the cell. Cytosolic proteins display little modification or processing compared to proteins that remain attached to the membranes of endoplasmic reticulum or the Golgi apparatus. Messenger RNA that encodes protein that will become a constituent of organelles or secretory products are formed on polysomes that are attached to endoplasmic reticulum. Such sheets of membrane in association with ribosomes are called rough endoplasmic reticulum. Secretory products typically undergo significant modification after translation. For example, neuropeptide transmitters are cleaved from polypeptide chains, in part, in the endoplasmic reticulum and the Golgi apparatus. Nuclear and mitochondrial proteins are encoded by the nucleus and are formed on free polysomes. The mechanism by which they are targeted to their proper organelle is called posttranslational importation. Specific receptors bind and translocate these proteins, and it is the recognition of the structural features of these proteins that allows for transport into the nucleus from the cytoplasm. In the processing of large proteins such as opioid peptides, more than one copy and different peptides are produced from the same precursor molecule. This precursor is referred to as a polyprotein because more than one active peptide is present.

64. The answer is D. (Kandel, 3rd Ed., pp. 40-41) The trigger zone for the initiation of impulses from a neuron includes a specialized region of the cell body, called the axon hillock, together with that section of the axon which adjoins this region — the initial segment. Other components of the neuron such as the dendrites and cell body receive inputs from afferent sources but are not capable of initiating impulses at these sites. The same is true concerning more distal aspects of the axon over which the impulse is conducted.

65. The answer is A. (Kandel, 3rd Ed. pp. 57-61; Carpenter and Sutin, 8th Ed., pp. 122-124) Transport of materials along an axon moves in both anterograde and retrograde directions. Anterograde transport involves both fast and slow transport systems. Transport in either direction utilizes microtubules as a vehicle or track by which the particles are transported. Among the particles transported down the axon from the cell body are newly synthesized membranous organelles including synaptic vesicles or their precursors which ultimately reach the axon terminals.

66. The answer is B. (Kandel, 3rd Ed., pp. 75-79) It is believed that different kinds of stimuli can function to open or close channels. For example, mechanical activation may lead to the opening of channels. Some channels (ligand-gated) are regulated by the noncovalent binding of chemical ligands such as neurotransmitters; others (electrically gated) are affected by changes in membrane voltage which cause a change in the conformation of the channel. Alternatively, relatively long-lasting changes may result when second messengers bind to the channel at which time there is protein phosphorylation mediated by protein kinases. Such modification of the channel can be reversed by dephosphorylation. In contrast, when a ligand-gated channel is exposed to prolonged, high concentrations of its ligand, it tends to become "refractory" (i.e., desensitized to the presence of that ligand).

67. The answer is A. (Kandel, 3rd Ed., pp. 68-79) Ion flux through ion channels is considered to be passive in nature and functions in the absence of any mechanism requiring energy metabolism. Cation channels are generally associated with membranes that are semipermeable to selective ions such as Na^+, K^+ or Cl^-. The electrochemical gradient is a function of two forces: (1) the chemical concentration gradient which is derived from the relative differences in the distributions of ions across the membrane, and (2) the electrical potential difference between the two sides of the membrane as a function of the distribution of the ionic charges. When ions may flow through channels, current varies as a function of concentration.

However, at high ionic concentration differences, a saturation phenomenon is observed that is due to resistance to flow through the channels.

68. The answer is A. (Kandel, 3rd Ed., pp. 95-97) The time and space constants represent passive properties of a neuron. The electrical equivalent circuit utilizes the concept that a membrane has both capacitive and resistive properties in parallel, in which case, the rising phase of a potential change is governed in part by the product of the resistance and capacitance of the membrane. The rising phase of a synaptic potential is governed by both active and passive properties of the membrane. However, the falling phase is regulated solely by the passive properties. As the time constant is increased, the probability of integration of converging synaptic signals is increased because such signals will be more likely to overlap in time (temporal summation).

69. The answer is C. (Kandel, 3rd Ed., pp. 82-85) The potential difference across the membrane is a result of the separation of charge and is called the resting membrane potential. Accordingly, the potential difference across the membrane is a direct function of the numbers of positive and negative charges on either side of the membrane. As the separation of charge across the membrane is reduced, the membrane is said to be depolarized. Conversely, as the separation of charge is increased, the membrane becomes hyperpolarized. In the latter case, the inside of the cell is made more negative with respect to the outside. If a cell has only a single channel in its membrane (such as for K^+), the gradients for the other ions become irrelevant and the membrane potential will approach the equilibrium potential for the single ion (K^+ in this example). There is a tendency for ions to leak down their electrochemical gradients from one side of the membrane to the other. In order for there to be a steady resting membrane potential, the gradients across the membrane must be held constant. Changes in ionic gradients are avoided, in spite of the leak, by the presence of an active Na^+/K^+ pump (a membrane protein) that moves Na^+ out of the cell and at the same time brings K^+ into the cell. Such a pumping mechanism requires energy because it is working against the electrochemical gradients of the two ions. The energy is derived from the hydrolysis of ATP.

70. The answer is B. (Kandel, 3rd Ed., pp. 97-100) The length constant is defined as:

$$\text{length constant} = R_m / R_a.$$

It is the distance along a fiber where a change in membrane potential produced by a given current decays to a value of approximately 1/3 of its original value. As can be seen from the equation, the length constant is directly proportional to the membrane resistance (R_m) and inversely related to the resistance of the cytoplasm within the fiber (i.e., axial resistance [R_a]). The membrane resistance is increased significantly through the process of myelination, which thus produces an increase in the value of the length constant. When the length constant along a dendrite is relatively large, it has the effect of increasing the efficiency of electrotonic conduction along the dendritic process as compared with a similar dendrite with a smaller length constant. In this manner, the synaptic potential along the dendrite distal to the synapse will be relatively larger in a dendrite that has a larger length constant than one that has a smaller length constant.

71. The answer is C. (Kandel, 3rd Ed., pp. 105-118) Sodium channels are rapidly opened following depolarization of the membrane. The rapid influx of ions results in a further depolarization of the membrane, which, in turn, can lead to an action potential. When the membrane is hyperpolarized, sodium channels are closed. Moreover, in the resting membrane, sodium channels are not activated. Tetraethylammonium is a drug that selectively blocks only potassium channels. Tetrodotoxin blocks sodium channels.

72. The answer is B. (Kandel, 3rd Ed., pp. 84-86, 88-91, 100-102, 105-108) Because the membrane is a leaky one, the sodium-potassium pump serves an important function in actively transporting ions from one side of the membrane to the other. The membrane is permeable to ions other than potassium, such as sodium and chloride. This fact is taken into consideration in the Goldman equation. This equation includes the distribution of all of these other ions in its formula for determining the value of membrane potential. Accordingly, the resting membrane potential is dependent upon the concentration of these other ions as well as potassium. While it is true that the Nernst equation considers the relative distribution of potassium ions across the membrane, this statement, in itself, does not explain why the equilibrium potential for potassium differs from the resting potential of the neuron. The statement that the Nernst equation does not take into account differences in temperature is false. But, again, even if that statement were true, it would nevertheless not account for the differences between the equilibrium potential for potassium and the resting potential of the neuron.

73. The answer is C. (Kandel, 3rd Ed. pp. 82-100) To solve the problem, use the Goldman equation which reduces to the Nernst equation:

$$\text{Equilibrium potential} \quad = \quad (RT / F) \times \ln [K_i] / [K_o]$$

$$-89.6 \quad = \quad 61 (\ln [K_i] - \ln [3])$$

$$-89.6 / 61 \quad = \quad \ln [K_i] - 0.48$$

$$1.47 \quad = \quad \ln [K_i] - 0.48$$

$$1.95 \quad = \quad \ln [K_i]$$

$$88.54 \quad = \quad K_i$$

74. The answer is C. (Kandel, 3rd Ed., pp. 82-100) If the bathing solution is brought to 88 mEq/L, the ionic concentrations outside and inside the membrane would be equal and, therefore, the membrane potential would be depolarized to zero.

75. The answer is A. (Kandel, pp. 82-100) Use the Goldman equation reduced to the Nernst equation. The resting membrane potential is -89.6 mV, $RT/F = 61$, the potassium concentration is 3 mEq/L, and K_i is calculated to be 88.54 mV. Therefore:

$$\text{Equilibrium Potential} \quad = \quad (RT / F) \times 61 \ln (K_o / K_i)$$

$$-89.6 - 12.1 \quad = \quad 61 \times \ln (K_o - 88.54)$$

$$-77.5 \quad = \quad 61 \times (\ln K_o - \ln 88.54)$$

$$-1.27 \quad = \quad \ln K_o - \ln 88.54$$

$$-1.27 - (-1.95) \quad = \quad \ln K_o$$

$$+0.68 \quad = \quad \ln K_o$$

$$4.79 \text{ mEq/L} \quad = \quad K_o$$

Therefore, the change in extracellular potassium would be:

$$4.79 - 3.00 \quad = \quad 1.79 \text{ mEq/L}.$$

76. The answer is A. (Kandel, 3rd Ed., pp. 82-100) In this situation the roles of sodium and chloride ions were not of central importance. Temporal summation also cannot account for these findings and is thus irrelevant to the question at hand. The depolarization of 12.1 mV can be attributed to an increase in the concentration of potassium in the intracellular cleft.

77. The answer is B. (Kandel, 3rd Ed., pp. 67-79; Guyton, 2nd Ed., pp. 60-61) The triggering mechanism for ligand-gating involves the selective binding of a particular molecule with the protein channel. This binding causes a conformational change of the channel protein that results in the movement of the channel back and forth which, in effect, opens or closes the channel. Neurotransmitters can regulate channels as a result of their binding properties. An example is the action of acetylcholine at the neuromuscular junction, which is capable of activating channels in the membrane of skeletal muscle. Most cation channels are selective for sodium, potassium, or calcium. Ion channels are composed of large membrane glycoproteins that vary widely in their molecular weights. In contrast to ligand-gating, other types of channels may be activated by changes in the electrical potential across the cell membrane, a process referred to as "voltage-gating."

78. The answer is A. (Kandel, 3rd Ed., pp. 105-118) In the late phase of the action potential, potassium channels become opened and potassium efflux produces a hyperpolarization of the membrane. During the repolarization of the membrane, sodium channels are closed (i.e., sodium inactivation). Recall that activation of sodium channels is associated with the generation of the action potential. Calcium has a strong electrochemical gradient that drives it into the cell, which coincides with the upstroke of the action potential. A number of different types of calcium gated potassium channels have been described that are activated during the action potential. Thus, it would appear that calcium influx during the action potential could generate opposing effects. On the one hand, calcium influx carries a positive charge into the cell which contributes to the depolarization of the membrane. On the other hand, calcium influx may help to open up more potassium channels, which contributes to an outward ionic flow of potassium causing repolarization of the membrane.

79. The answer is E. (Kandel, pp. 88-91, 96-102) To understand how an inhibitory transmitter can actually cause a partial depolarization of the membrane, refer to the Goldman equation. The release (or application) of an inhibitory transmitter will serve to open specific ion channels, notably those of potassium. If the membrane is artificially hyperpolarized to – 120 mV, the opening of the potassium channel will lead to a redistribution of the ions across the membrane to a normal level. If the normal equilibrium potential for potassium is approximately -75 mV, then, application of an inhibitory transmitter (that typically functions by opening potassium channels) will result in a redistribution of potassium ions towards the potassium equilibrium potential (i.e., -75 mV). Consequently, the membrane potential will be reduced (i.e., depolarized) from -120 mV to a value close to -75 mV. Other possible answers are clearly incorrect. Inhibitory transmitters normally function to hyperpolarize the membrane. Postsynaptic membranes may either be depolarized or hyperpolarized, depending upon the nature of the transmitter and receptor complex present at the synapse. Since the influx of calcium during the depolarization phase of the action potential leads to opposing effects, activation of this channel cannot account for the observed effects. Inactivation of sodium channels would not result in a depolarization of the membrane, but, instead, may contribute to the hyperpolarization of the membrane.

The Synapse

DIRECTIONS: Each group of questions below consists of lettered headings followed by a set of numbered items. For each numbered item select the **one** lettered heading with which it is **most** closely associated. Each lettered item may be used **once, more than once, or not at all**.

Questions 80 - 85

     (A) resting potential

     (B) action potential

     (C) receptor potential

     (D) electrical postsynaptic potentials

     (E) increased-conductance postsynaptic potentials

     (F) decreased-conductance postsynaptic potentials

80. all or none, approximately 100 mV

81. a relatively steady voltage, which varies from cell to cell and ranging from − 35 to − 90 mV

82. a graded, fast potential, lasting from several milliseconds to seconds, resulting from a chemical transmitter binding to a receptor to produce either an EPSP that depends upon a single class of channels for sodium and potassium or an IPSP that is dependent upon chloride or potassium conductance

83. a graded, slow potential, lasting from seconds to minutes; contributes to the amplitude and duration of the action potential; it involves a chemical transmitter and an intracellular messenger for the closure of single-ion channels

84. activated by a sensory stimulus, this potential lasts for several milliseconds, is graded, and involves a single channel for both sodium and potassium ions

85. characterized by the passive spread of a presynaptic current across a gap junction and activated by changes in voltage, pH, or calcium ion levels

Questions 86- 89

(A) axodendritic synapse

(B) axoaxonic synapse

(C) axosomatic synapse

(D) somasomatic synapse

(E) dendrodendritric synapse

86. these synapses are frequently found to be excitatory

87. these synapses are frequently found to be inhibitory

88. at these synapses, the neuron is regulated as a result of the modulation of the quantity of transmitter released

89. this type of synapse is characteristic of the one present between the basket and Purkinje cells of the cerebellum

---

DIRECTIONS: Each question below contains five suggested responses. Select the one best response to each question.

90. All of the following statements concerning electrical synapses are true EXCEPT:

(A) The zone connecting the two neurons is referred to as a gap junction.

(B) In most cases, electrical synapses are considered rectifying.

(C) Typically, current may flow equally well from the postsynaptic cell into the presynaptic cell as it does from the presynaptic cell into the postsynaptic cell.

(D) The structure of the synapse may be viewed as a pair of cylinders or hemi-channels, one on the presynaptic and the other on the postsynaptic side.

(E) Electrical transmission may be modulated by the presence of intracellular calcium.

91. All of the following statements concerning chemical synapses are correct EXCEPT:

(A) Presynaptic terminals contain many vesicles that are normally filled with a chemical neurotransmitter.

(B) The postsynaptic receptor determines whether or not a transmitter will bind to a receptor molecule on the postsynaptic cell.

(C) The receptors are proteins.

(D) Receptors can provide a gating function with respect to a given ion channel.

(E) The mechanism of indirect gating of ions normally does not involve the activation of G-proteins.

92. Concerning the neuromuscular junction, all of the following are correct EXCEPT:

(A) the membrane of the muscle cell in the end plate region contains extensive numbers of voltage-gated sodium channels

(B) the end plate potential is a result of the interaction of acetylcholine (ACh), released from the nerve terminal, with the ACh receptor in the muscle membrane

(C) ACh is rapidly removed from the synaptic cleft through hydrolysis by acetylcholinesterase as well as by diffusion

(D) at the end plate, separate transmitter-gated channels for sodium and potassium, activated by ACh, are responsible for the synaptic potential

(E) the arrival of an action potential at the nerve terminal opens many calcium channels

93. Gamma-aminobutyric acid (GABA) and glycine share all of the following properties EXCEPT?

(A) both are known to have inhibitory as well as excitatory properties

(B) both, acting on different receptors, regulate a similar chloride channel

(C) both utilize receptors that are transmembrane proteins

(D) both have channels that produce electrical signals because ions move down their electrochemical gradients within their respective channels

(E) both are found in the spinal cord

94. N-methyl-D-aspartate (NMDA), kainate, and quisqualate all act on which of the following receptors:

(A) Gamma aminobutyric acid receptors

(B) excitatory amino acid receptors

(C) adrenergic receptors

(D) opioid receptors

(E) dopamine receptors

95. Characteristics of the N-methyl-D-aspartate (NMDA) receptor include all of the following EXCEPT:

(A) it controls a high conductance cation channel

(B) the NMDA channel is easily blocked by the presence of magnesium

(C) the NMDA channel has voltage-gating properties

(D) excessive amounts of glutamate, acting through NMDA receptors, may cause neuronal cell death

(E) current flow is blocked in the presence of glutamate, leading to hyperpolarization of the cell

96. Which of the following is a second messenger system directly activated by the binding of norepinephrine to a beta-adrenergic receptor:

(A) inositol 1,4,5-triphosphate (IP3)

(B) cyclic AMP

(C) diacylglycerol (DAG)

(D) arachidonic acid

(E) prostaglandins

97. Inhibition at the synapse is governed by:

(A) chloride and sodium

(B) chloride and potassium

(C) potassium and sodium

(D) sodium and calcium

(E) sodium only

98. Which of the following statements is appropriate to second messengers within neurons:

(A) They have little effect upon the activity of ion channels.

(B) They can regulate gene expression which could lead to neuronal growth and the synthesis of new proteins.

(C) They have little effect upon the opening or closing of ion channels.

(D) They have little effect upon receptors.

(E) They are directly involved in the gating of sodium channels by NMDA receptors.

99. The release of transmitter is directly governed by:

(A) sodium influx

(B) sodium efflux

(C) potassium influx

(D) potassium efflux

(E) calcium influx

100. All of the following statements concerning synaptic connections on presynaptic terminals are correct EXCEPT:

(A) They occur when one axon contacts the axon terminal of another cell.

(B) They can inhibit but cannot facilitate transmitter release.

(C) Inhibition is generated by a presynaptic neuron when it depresses the calcium current in the terminal of a second presynaptic neuron.

(D) Axo-axonic synapses are typically present in sensory relay nuclei.

(E) Presynaptic inhibition also involves increased conductances of chloride and potassium.

The Synapse

Answers

80-85. The answers are 80-B, 81-A, 82-E, 83-F, 84-C, 85-D. (Kandel, 3rd Ed., pp. 123-172) The action potential (B) is characterized by an all or none response in which the overshoot may reach an amplitude of up to 100 mV. The mechanism involves separate ion channels for sodium and potassium. The resting potential (A) is characterized by a relatively steady potential, usually in the region of -70 mV, but which may range from -35 to -70 mV. This potential is mainly dependent upon potassium and chloride channels. Increased-conductance postsynaptic potentials (E) are fast, graded potentials lasting from several milliseconds to several seconds. If the potential is an EPSP, it depends upon a single class of ligand-gated channels for sodium and potassium. If the response is an IPSP, then it depends upon ligand-gated channels for potassium and chloride. Decreased-conductance postsynaptic potentials (F) are mediated by a chemical transmitter or intracellular messenger to produce a graded, slow potential, lasting from seconds to minutes. The response is related to a closure of sodium, potassium, or chloride channels. Receptor potentials (C) result from the application of a sensory stimulus that produces a fast, graded potential that involves a single class of channels for both sodium and potassium. Electrical postsynaptic potentials (D) involve the passive spread of current across a gap junction that is permeable to a variety of small ions. The stimulus for such activation may either be a change in voltage, pH, or intracellular calcium.

86-89. The answers are 86-A, 87-C, 88-B, 89-C. (Kandel, 3rd Ed, pp. 166-172, 626-632) The overwhelming number of excitatory synapses are observed to be axodendritic (A). The presynaptic axon may synapse upon either the dendritic spine or the dendritic trunk. In contrast, axon terminals that make synaptic contact with the soma (C) of postsynaptic cells are frequently observed to be inhibitory. A classic example of this is in the cerebellar cortex where an interneuron (basket cell) makes synaptic contact with the soma of the Purkinje cell. Activation of the basket cell results in subsequent inhibition of the Purkinje cell. Axoaxonic synapses are formed when an axon terminal comes into synaptic contact with another axon. While axoaxonic synapses have no direct effect upon the trigger zone of the postsynaptic cell, they affect that cell's functioning indirectly by modulating the amount of transmitter released from its axon terminals. Dendrodendritic synapses have been identified in the olfactory bulb and have been shown to be inhibitory. They are not found with any frequency in any other region of the central nervous system.

The Synapse 33

90. The answer is B. (Kandel, 3rd Ed., pp. 123-130) The apposition of the two neuronal elements that form an electrical synapse is called a gap junction and contains bridges that are referred to as gap junction channels. It is through these channels that ionic current flows for electrical transmission. Gap junctions are separated by very small spaces, extending only a distance of approximately 3.5 nm. Most electrical synapses are nonrectifying. Thus, current flow is bidirectional. Current that is injected into a presynaptic cell will depolarize that cell, and the current will also flow into the postsynaptic cell and depolarize it. Because the coupling mechanism associated with nonrectifying synapses is symmetrical, current will flow equally well from either cell to the other and depolarization of either cell will occur. Gap junctions consist of a pair of cylinders that help to form channels, one on the presynaptic side and the other on the postsynaptic side. The cylinders meet in the gap forming a communicating channel between the two cells. The channel thus formed is referred to as a connexon and is composed of 6 identical subunits called connexins. The role of the connexin is to recognize the other 5 protein subunits in order to form an effective hemi-channel and to recognize its counterpart on the postsynaptic side. Transmission can be modulated by a number of factors, which include the presence of intracellular calcium and changes in intracellular pH. The presence of these factors likely contribute to the closing of the gap junction channels.

91. The answer is E. (Kandel, 3rd Ed., pp. 131-134) The presynaptic terminals of chemical synapses typically contain synaptic vesicles. The vesicles may be round or flat, and filled or empty. They are typically filled with a neurotransmitter that is released onto the synaptic cleft. The receptive process on the postsynaptic region — i.e., the postsynaptic receptor — takes on a very important function. The binding of the transmitter to the receptor molecule is determined by this receptor, which is a membrane spanning protein. Perhaps the most significant feature of the receptor is that it serves a gating function for particular ions. It can do this either directly, if it is part of the ion channel, or indirectly, by activating a G-protein, that, in turn, activates a second messenger system. This process results in a modulation of the ion channel's activity. In particular, the G-protein stimulates adenylate cyclase, converting ATP to cAMP. In turn, cAMP induces activation of cAMP dependent protein kinase, which modulates channels by phosphorylating the channel protein or some other protein that works on that channel.

92. The answer is D. (Kandel, 3rd Ed., pp. 135-145; Guyton 2nd Ed., pp. 308-311) There are extensive numbers of voltage-gated sodium channels present along the membrane of the muscle cell end-plate region. These channels are critical for the generation of action potentials. While potassium ions are small enough to pass through an acetylcholine channel, very few of them actually do because of the negative potential on the inside of the cell membrane. The following sequence of events comprises the steps that lead to a muscle action potential: when a motor nerve action potential reaches the region of the presynaptic terminals, it causes many calcium channels to open and the inward calcium current facilitates the release of acetylcholine from the presynaptic terminal. Acetylcholine release and subsequent binding to ACh receptors on the postsynaptic membrane leads to the opening of channels which permit the passage of sodium ions to the inside of the muscle cell. The sudden increase in positive charges inside the cell produces a local potential called the end-plate potential. The muscle action potential is then initiated by the end-plate potential, which results in a muscle contraction. The acetylcholine released into the synaptic cleft is removed by two mechanisms: (1) diffusion away from the synaptic cleft so that it cannot act upon the muscle membrane (this accounts for only a small percentage); and (2) through hydrolysis by the enzyme acetylcholinesterase, which accounts for the removal of most of the acetylcholine.

93. The answer is A. (Kandel, 3rd Ed., pp. 160-170) Both GABA and glycine are inhibitory transmitters found in the spinal cord and elsewhere in the central nervous system. Accordingly, they both act on a similar chloride channel, which, when activated, permits this ion to enter the cell and make it more negative (i.e., hyperpolarize the cell). Each of the channels is formed from a transmembrane protein. It contains a transmitter binding site on the outer side of the membrane, and its conducting pore is embedded in the cell membrane. Another feature — that both channels produce electrical signals as a result of the movement of ions down their electrochemical gradients within their channels — is a feature common to both excitatory and inhibitory transmitters.

94. The answer is B. (Kandel, 3rd Ed., pp. 157-160) NMDA, kainate, and quisqualate act upon excitatory amino acid receptors. The NMDA receptor differs from the other types of receptors in that it is blocked by Mg^{++} and controls a cation channel permeable to calcium, sodium and potassium. Pharmacologically, NMDA receptors can blocked by 2-amino-5 phosphonovaleric acid. The quisqualate receptor is activated by quisqualic acid; it has a high affinity for L-glutamate and a- amino-hydroxy-5-methyl-4-isoxazolepropionic acid (AMPA). The kainate receptor is activated by kainic acid. It regulates a channel that is permeable to sodium and potassium, binds AMPA, and is important in the process of excitotoxicity.

95. The answer is E. (Kandel, 3rd Ed., pp. 152-160) The NMDA receptor regulates a channel permeable to several cations which include calcium, sodium, and potassium. This channel, however, is easily blocked by magnesium. In fact, it requires a significant depolarization of the membrane in order for magnesium to be exuded from the channel so that sodium and calcium can enter the cell. One of the unusual features of this transmitter-gated channel is that it is also gated by voltage. Thus, conductance reaches its peak when both glutamate is present and the cell is depolarized. High concentrations of glutamate could result in death of the cell. This may be due to an unusually large influx of calcium through NMDA activated channels. The calcium might activate proteases, resulting in the formation of free radicals that could be toxic to the cell.

96. The answer is B. (Kandel, 3rd Ed., pp. 173-176) When norepinephrine reaches a beta-adrenergic receptor, a G-protein activates adenyl cyclase which generates a second messenger, cyclic AMP from ATP. Cyclic AMP activates a cyclic AMP-dependent kinase that alters the conformation of regulatory subunits of other kinases. This frees catalytic subunits to phosphorylate specific proteins which, in turn, leads to the cellular response. IP_3 and DAG are associated with the transmitter acetylcholine which binds to muscarinic receptors, and arachidonic acid is linked to histamine which binds to histamine receptors. Prostaglandins are metabolites of arachidonic acid.

97. The answer is B. (Kandel, 3rd Ed., pp. 160-168) In neurons within the CNS, an inhibitory transmitter will open chloride channels. In addition, second messengers may also mediate inhibition. It is likely that they do so by opening potassium channels. When a chloride channel is opened, it will lead to movement of this ion down its concentration gradient and into the cell. This will make the cell more negative (i.e., hyperpolarized). At the same time, there will be an efflux of potassium, which will also produce hyperpolarization of the cell because positive charges are now being removed. On the other hand, sodium and calcium influx are associated with depolarization of the cell.

98. The answer is B. (Kandel, 3rd Ed., pp. 180-192) Second messenger kinases can lead to the phosphorylation of ion channel proteins. Such a process can lead to either the closing of a previously open ion channel or opening of a previously closed channel. For example, norepinephrine acts through cyclic AMP to close the potassium channel resulting in an increase in excitability. Second messengers can phosphorylate transcriptional regulatory proteins and thus alter gene expression. In particular, existing proteins may be altered and new proteins may be synthesized. Moreover, such effects may generate other alterations such as the induction of neuronal growth. Second messengers can also interact directly with an ion channel to cause it to open or close (in the absence of a protein kinase). They also can produce a level of desensitization in receptors which is a function of the extent of phosphorylation. The direct gating of ion channels by NMDA receptors is an example of a process that does not immediately involve a second messenger.

99. The answer is E. (Kandel, 3rd Ed., pp. 194-211) Experimental methods permit evaluation of the relative contributions of different ions in the regulation of transmitter release. Neither tetrodotoxin, which blocks voltage-gated sodium channels, nor tetraethylammonium, which blocks voltage-gated potassium channels, will block the generation of a postsynaptic potential when the presynaptic cell is artificially depolarized. In contrast, presynaptic calcium influx triggers the release of transmitter and results in a postsynaptic potential. Moreover, when presynaptic calcium influx is blocked, no postsynaptic potential is produced. Action potentials at the presynaptic axon terminals open up calcium channels permitting calcium influx. This event helps move synaptic vesicles to active sites as actin filaments (which anchor the vesicles) are dissolved.

100. The answer is B. (Kandel, 3rd Ed., Ch. 13, pp. 207-210) Axoaxonic synapses, most commonly present in sensory relay nuclei, are found when axon terminals of one neuron make synaptic contact with axon terminals of a second neuron which is also in contact with a (third) postsynaptic cell. Axoaxonic synapses may either inhibit or facilitate transmitter release by the target axon. In presynaptic facilitation, the facilitating neuron reduces potassium current in the axon terminal of the target neuron. This can increase the duration of action potentials and associated calcium current leading to increased transmitter release by the target axon. In presynaptic inhibition, there is a closure of calcium channels (causing a decrease in calcium influx) and an increase in both potassium and chloride conductances resulting in a smaller depolarization and a further reduction in calcium influx.

Neurotransmitters

DIRECTIONS: The questions below consist of lettered headings followed by a set of numbered items. For each numbered item select the **one** heading with which it is **most** closely associated. Each lettered heading may be used **once, more than once, or not at all.**

Questions 101-111

(A) tyrosine

(B) serotonin

(C) phenylalanine

(D) dihydroxyphenylalanine (L-DOPA)

(E) dopamine beta hydroxylase

(F) dopamine

(G) norepinephrine

(H) tryptophan hydroxylase

(I) choline acetyltransferase

(J) monoamine oxidase

(K) p-chlorophenylalanine

(L) phenylethanolamine-N-methyl transferase

(M) tyrosine hydroxylase

101. An immediate precursor of dopamine

102. rate limiting enzyme in the biosynthesis of serotonin

103. enzyme converting dopamine to norepinephrine

104. amino acid precursor of dihydroxyphenylalanine (L-DOPA)

105. immediate precursor of epinephrine

106. immediate precursor of norepinephrine

107. transmitter destroyed by 5,7-dihydroxytryptamine (5,7-DHT)

108. enzyme converting norepinephrine to epinephrine

109. depletes brain serotonin

110. involved in metabolic degredation of catecholamines

111. first enzyme involved in the biosynthesis of catecholamines

DIRECTIONS: The questions below consist of lettered headings followed by a set of numbered items. For each numbered item select the **one** heading with which it is **most** closely associated. Each lettered heading may be used **once, more than once, or not at all.**

Questions 112-121

      (A) norepinephrine

      (B) somatostatin

      (C) cholecystokinin

      (D) dopamine

      (E) serotonin

      (F) oxytocin

      (G) gamma-aminobutyric acid (GABA)

      (H) glycine

      (I) enkephalins

      (J) substance P

      (K) glutamate

      (L) acetylcholine

112. an inhibitory interneuron in the spinal cord

113. present in raphe neurons of the pons and caudal midbrain

114. present in the ventral tegmental and interpeduncular neurons of the midbrain

115. present in the locus ceruleus of the pons

116. present in the pars compacta of the substantia nigra

117. transmitter of cortical neurons that project to the neostriatum

118. a transmitter generally regarded as inhibitory, synthesized exclusively in the cell body, and present in high concentrations in the midbrain periaqueductal gray where it is believed to modulate pain impulses

119. found in high concentrations within the nucleus basalis of the rostral forebrain which supplies the cerebral cortex

120. an excitatory transmitter that is released from endings of primary sensory afferents of the spinal cord

121. directly antagonized by bicuculline and benzodiazepines are sometimes referred to as agonists for this transmitter

Questions: 122-138

(A) 5-hydroxytryptamine-2 (5-HT$_2$) agonist

(B) 5-hydroxytryptamine-1 (5-HT$_1$) agonist

(C) N-methyl-D-aspartate (NMDA) antagonist

(D) excitatory amino acid receptor

(E) gamma-aminobutyric acid-B (GABA$_B$) agonist

(F) gamma-aminobutyric acid-A (GABA$_A$) antagonist

(G) opiate kappa agonist

(H) opiate mu agonist

(I) 5-HT$_2$ antagonist

(J) dopamine D$_2$ antagonist

(K) alpha-2 receptor antagonist

(L) muscarinic agonist

(M) alpha-2 receptor agonist

(N) alpha-1 receptor antagonist

(O) nicotinic antagonist

(P) muscarinic antagonist

(Q) beta-1 adrenergic antagonist

(R) opiate antagonist

122. yohimbine

123. clonidine

124. prazosin

125. metoprolol

126. sulpiride

127. oxotremorine

128. morphine

129. naloxone

130. dynorphin

131. quinuclidinyl benzilate (QNB)

132. ketanserin

133. bicuculline

134. baclofen

135. N-methyl-D-aspartate (NMDA)

136. quisqualate

137. kainate

138. alpha-Bungarotoxin

DIRECTIONS: Each question below contains five suggested responses. Select the one best response to each question.

139. The biochemical sequence involved in synaptic transmission is:

(A) transmitter synthesis —> binding of transmitter to postsynaptic receptor —> release of transmitter into synaptic cleft —> destruction of transmitter

(B) transmitter synthesis —> release of transmitter into synaptic cleft —> binding of transmitter to postsynaptic receptor —> removal of transmitter

(C) transmitter synthesis —> breakdown of calcium channels —> binding of transmitter to postsynaptic receptor —> destruction of receptor

(D) breakdown of calcium channels —> transmitter synthesis —> binding of transmitter to postsynaptic receptor —> removal of transmitter

(E) breakdown of calcium channels —> transmitter synthesis —> binding of transmitter to presynaptic receptor —> reuptake of transmitter

140. All of the following are amino acids or amino acid derived transmitters EXCEPT:

(A) gamma-aminobutyric acid (GABA)

(B) glycine

(C) acetylcholine

(D) glutamate

(E) aspartate

141. All of the following statements about glutamate in the brain are true EXCEPT:

(A) Glutamate is distributed over wide areas within the central nervous system.

(B) Glutamate is an amino acid utilized for protein synthesis.

(C) Glutamate is known to be an inhibitory transmitter in the ventromedial hypothalamus.

(D) Glutamate is a precursor of GABA.

(E) When glutamate is applied iontophoretically onto neurons of the caudate nucleus, excitation will occur.

142. Monoamines differ from neuroactive peptides in which of the following ways:

(A) monoamines are synthesized only in the cell body of neurons

(B) synthesis (in monoamines) is governed by messenger RNA on ribosomes which is not true for neuroactive peptides

(C) monoamines are generally synthesized as part of a larger precursor molecule called a prohormone

(D) monoamine neurons are generally regarded as having only excitatory properties, while peptides are inhibitory

(E) monoamine neurons are principally found within brainstem nuclei, while peptide-containing neurons are found throughout the brain

143. An enzyme that is directly responsible for the degradation of norepinephrine is:

(A) tryptophan hydroxylase

(B) tyrosine hydroxylase

(C) dopamine beta-hydroxylase

(D) catechol-O-methyltransferase

(E) choline acetyltransferase

144. All of the following are usually classified as excitatory transmitters EXCEPT:

(A) glutamate

(B) acetylcholine

(C) substance P

(D) leucine

(E) aspartate

145. All of the following statements concerning neuroactive peptides are correct EXCEPT:

(A) Thyrotropin-releasing hormone (TRH) and gonadotropin-releasing hormone (GnRH) are examples of neuroactive peptides present in the hypothalamus.

(B) Normally, gastrointestinal peptides such as cholycystokinin are not present in the central nervous system (CNS) and presumably do not act via the CNS to modify physiological processes.

(C) Neuropeptides are often found to be colocalized with other transmitter substances such as the monoamines.

(D) Neuropeptides can be identified anatomically with selective immunochemical staining procedures.

(E) Neuropeptides are distributed over wide areas of the CNS.

146. All of the following are normally classified as inhibitory compounds EXCEPT:

(A) glycine

(B) gamma-aminobutyric acid (GABA)

(C) enkephalin

(D) muscimol

(E) strychnine

147. All of the following are drugs that affect central cholinergic synapses EXCEPT:

(A) atropine

(B) scopolamine

(C) haloperidol

(D) physostigmine

(E) hemicholinium

148. Phenylketonuria is a disease that occurs when:

(A) ineffective enzyme activity leads to phenylalanine levels that are abnormally high

(B) phenylalanine is converted to tyrosine in excessive amounts, leading to abnormal levels of catecholamines in the brain

(C) tyrosine cannot be converted to DOPA

(D) dopamine cannot be converted to norepinephrine

(E) catecholamine levels remain extremely high as a result of the failure of monoamine oxidase to degrade norepinephrine and dopamine

149. A long-lasting depletion of norepinephrine can be produced by administration of:

(A) amphetamine

(B) apomorphine

(C) clonidine

(D) reserpine

(E) yohimbine

150. In a recent study, it was observed that when catecholamines released from its terminal endings, further release of this transmitter is temporarily blocked. A similar attenuation of release of catecholamine was noted when an agonist was administered to the preparation. These results are best understood in terms of:

(A) the presence of a GABAergic neuron at the synapse

(B) postsynaptic inhibition

(C) the presence of presynaptic autoreceptors

(D) destruction of the catecholamine cell body

(E) collateral inhibition

151. All of the following statements about synaptic vesicles are true EXCEPT:

(A) Transmitters such as catecholamines are passively taken up into synaptic vesicles along an osmotic gradient.

(B) Synaptic vesicles are directly involved in the release of transmitter by an exocytotic process.

(C) Synaptic vesicles move from the Golgi apparatus down the axon to the axon terminal where they join a large pool of other vesicles.

(D) The membranes of synaptic vesicles contain specific proteins which carry out distinct functions such as the mobilization of vesicles into docking sites at the synaptic membrane.

(E) Synaptic vesicles are generally recycled.

152. Removal of norepinephrine from the region of the synaptic cleft may be achieved by which of the following mechanisms:

(A) reuptake

(B) enzymatic degradation

(C) diffusion

(D) a combination of enzymatic degradation and diffusion

(E) a combination of enzymatic degradation, diffusion, and reuptake

153. All of the following statements concerning myasthenia gravis are true EXCEPT:

(A) The likelihood that transmission will take place at the neuromuscular junction is reduced because there are morphological changes at the junction.

(B) The amplitude of the end-plate potential of the myasthenic patient is the same as that of a normal individual.

(C) Myasthenia gravis results from an autoimmune reaction directed against the acetylcholine receptor.

(D) The normal pattern and rate of destruction of acetylcholine receptors is significantly increased in myasthenic patients.

(E) One successful approach to therapeutic treatment of this disorder is thymectomy.

154. All of the following statements concerning the motor unit are true EXCEPT:

(A) A motor unit is defined as a motor neuron and the group of muscle fibers innervated by that motor neuron.

(B) A muscle is said to have atrophied when it has become weak and "wasted away."

(C) Muscle atrophy is a necessary consequence of an upper motor neuron disorder.

(D) Fasciculations are characterized by spontaneous activity within a single motor uni,t while fibrillations involve spontaneous activity within single muscle fibers.

(E) Demyelinating diseases result in a lowering of nerve conduction velocities.

Neurotransmitters

Answers

101-111. The answers are: 101-D, 102-H, 103-E, 104-A, 105-G, 106-F, 107-B, 108-L, 109-K, 110-J, 111-M. (Cooper, 6th Ed., pp. 225-227, 236, 255, 257, 290, 298-299, 324, 341; Kandel, 3rd Ed., pp. 215-217) The biosynthesis of catecholamines includes the following steps: tyrosine (A) is converted into dihydroxyphenylalanine (L-DOPA) (D) by tyrosine hydroxylase (M). L-DOPA is then decarboxylated by a decarboxylase to form dopamine (and CO_2). The conversion of dopamine (F) to norepinephrine is accomplished by the action of the enzyme dopamine beta hydroxylase (E). Finally, norepinephrine (G) is converted to epinephrine by the enzyme phenylethanolamine-N-methyl transferase (L). Catecholamines are metabolically degraded by monoamine oxidase (J) and catechol-O-methyltransferase. The rate-limiting enzyme in the biosynthesis of serotonin is tryptophan hydroxylase (H). In this process, tryptophan is converted to 5-hydroxytrypophan by tryptophan hydroxylase and by 5-hydroxytryptophan decarboxylase into serotonin. The drug, p-chlorophenylalanine (K), has been used experimentally to deplete serotonin levels in the brain. In addition, 5,7-dihydroxytryptamine (5,7-DHT) is a neurotoxic compound that selectively destroys serotonin (B) neurons.

112-121. The answers are: 112-H (or G), 113-E, 114-D, 115-A, 116-D, 117-K, 118-I, 119-L, 120J, 121-G. (Kandel, 3rd Ed., pp. 162, 213-224, 395-398, 649-656, 683-698; Cooper, 6th Ed., pp. 152-153, 169, 184-185, 263, 302-303, 314-315, 349, 394-395, 408-409) Glycine (H) has been identified by electrophysiological methods as an inhibitory transmitter of spinal interneurons. Other studies have indicated that it also may be an inhibitory transmitter in the retina. Serotonin (E) neurons are localized to clusters of cells along the midline of the pons and midbrain. These clusters are known as raphe nuclei and constitute the primary, if not exclusive, source of serotonin to both the hindbrain and the forebrain. The majority of dopamine (D) neurons are localized in the ventral tegmental area, interpeduncular nucleus, and pars compacta of the substantia nigra. Fibers from the ventral tegmental area and interpeduncular nucleus supply most of the forebrain including the cortex, while dopamine neurons from the substantia nigra supply the striatum. Much of the norepinephrine (A) that reaches the forebrain arises from neurons located in a region of the upper pons called the locus ceruleus. Many of the descending fibers from the cerebral cortex utilize glutamate (K) as their transmitter. This is especially true for cortical fibers that supply the neostriatum. Enkephalin (I) neurons play an important role in the regulation of ascending pain inputs. Significant modulation takes place at the level of the midbrain periaqueductal gray where enkephalins are present in high concentrations and are generally inhibitory. Enkephalins are synthesized exclusively in the cell body and are then transported down the axon to the terminals. Acetylcholine (L) is generally regarded as an excitatory transmitter and is present over wide areas of the central nervous system (CNS). Of particular significance is the nucleus basalis of the rostral forebrain which contains high concentrations of cholinergic neurons that supply the cerebral cortex. Loss of these cholinergic neurons has been implicated in the development of Alzheimer's disease. Substance P (J) is an excitatory transmitter that is present over wide areas of the CNS. In particular, it has been identified as the transmitter of primary sensory afferents which terminate in the dorsal horn of the spinal cord. Gamma-aminobutyric acid (GABA) (G) is an inhibitory transmitter. Direct antagonists for this transmitter (e.g., bicuculline) have been developed. Benzodiazepines potentiate the action of tonically released GABA by displacing an endogenous inhibitor of receptor binding. Benzodiazepines may do this by modifying the affinity of GABA for its own receptor or by coupling the GABA receptor to the chloride ion channel.

122-138. The answers are: 122-K, 123-M, 124-N, 125-Q, 126-J, 127-P, 128-H, 129-R, 130-G, 131-L, 132-I, 133-F, 134-E, 135D, 136-D, 137-D, 138-O. (Cooper, 6th Ed., pp. 181, 210, 216, 275-276, 302-303, 354-356, 401-404) For many of the transmitters that have been studied in recent years, different receptor subtypes have been identified for which specific agonist and antagonist compounds have been developed. The significance of the development of these compounds is that they can be used as experimental tools to determine the physiological role of different receptors. They have also been used effectively in the treatment of various disorders. For norepinephrine, the following receptors have been identified: alpha-1, alpha-2, beta-1, and beta-2. Yohimbine is a selective alpha-2 antagonist; clonidine, a selective alpha-2 agonist; prazosin, an alpha-1 antagonist; and metoprolol, a beta-1 receptor antagonist. For dopamine, D_1 and D_2 receptors have been identified. Several highly selective compounds have been produced in recent years. As an example, sulpiride is characterized as a selective D_2 antagonist. A number of different serotonin receptor subtypes have also been identified. As an illustration, ketanserin is classified as a preferential 5-hydroxytryptamine-2 (5-HT$_2$) receptor antagonist. Different opiate receptors have also been identifed: μ, δ, κ, and σ receptors. Morphine has μ agonist properties; dynorphin is a κ agonist and naloxone is a non-specific antagonist that preferentially acts upon μ receptors. Two different classes of cholinergic receptors have been identified — muscarinic and nicotinic receptors. Quinuclidinyl benzilate (QNB) is a selective muscarinic antagonist, α-Bungarotoxin is a selective nicotinic antagonist, and oxotremorine is a selective muscarinic agonist. With respect to gamma-aminobutyric acid (GABA), a variety of receptor subtypes is known. Bicuculline acts as a GABA$_A$ antagonist and baclofen is a selective GABA$_B$ agonist. With respect to excitatory amino acids, three different classes of receptors have been identified — these include N-methyl-D-aspartate (NMDA), quisqualate, and kainate receptors. While selective antagonists for NMDA are available, specific antagonists for each of the other receptors have yet to be established. However, drugs are available that will collectively block quisqualate and kainate receptors but not NMDA receptors.

139. The correct answer is B. (Kandel, 3rd Ed., pp. 213-215) Initially, final synthesis of the transmitter takes place in the neuron. The transmitter is then present in the presynaptic terminal and is released into the synaptic cleft where it binds to the postynaptic receptor. Finally, it is removed from the synaptic cleft or destroyed. Recall also that a necessary stimulus for the release of transmitter is the influx of calcium (through calcium channels) into the synaptic terminal.

140. The answer is C. (Kandel, 3rd Ed., pp. 214-218) Gamma-aminobutyric acid GABA, glycine, glutamate, and aspartate are all amino acids. In contrast, acetylcholine is synthesized from acetyl coenzyme A plus choline.

141. The answer is C. (Kandel, 3rd Ed., pp. 215-218; Cooper, 6th Ed., pp. 173-185) Glutamate has a number of different functions within the central nervous system (CNS). It plays an important role in neural synthesis of proteins and peptides – it is a precursor in the biosynthesis of GABA. It is widely distributed throughout the CNS (with unequal regional distributions) and is known to be an excitatory transmitter. Infusion of glutamate onto most, if not all, cells in the CNS will result in their excitation.

142. The answer is E. (Kandel, 3rd Ed., pp. 217-221; Cooper, 6th Ed., pp. 382-385, 391-394) Peptides differ from other neurotransmitters in several ways. Monoamines can be formed in all parts of the neuron with the completion of synthesis at the nerve terminal. In contrast, peptides are formed as a result of messenger RNA that is directed upon ribosomes, thus limiting the site of synthesis to the cell body where the processing is accomplished by the endoplasmic reticulum and Golgi apparatus. Typically, different neuroactive peptides are cleaved from a single, much larger molecule, called a prohormone that has no biological activity. The active peptide is cleaved by specific peptidases and is ultimately transported down the axon to the nerve terminal. In addition, the overwhelming majority of monoamine neurons are situated in the brainstem, while neuroactive peptides can be found over widespread regions of both the brainstem and forebrain, and, in particular, limbic structures. Both monoamines and peptides may display inhibitory as well as excitatory properties. For example, enkephalins are generally inhibitory, while substance P neurons are excitatory. Monoamine neurons may have excitatory effects in one region of the brain and inhibitory effects in another region.

143. The answer is D. (Kandel, 3rd Ed., pp. 213-221; Cooper, 6th Ed., pp. 224-229, 244-246) Tryptophan hydroxylase, tyrosine hydroxylase, and choline acetyltransferase are enzymes that are critical for the biosynthesis of serotonin, catecholamines, and acetylcholine, respectively. Dopamine beta-hydroxylase converts dopamine to norepinephrine. Catechol-O-methyltransferase and monoamine oxidase are critical for the metabolic degradation of catecholamines.

144. The answer is D. (Cooper, 6th Ed., pp. 168-169, 201-202, 207-208, 394-396) Electrophysiological and pharmacological studies have demonstrated that iontophoretic application of glutamate and aspartate onto cells of the central nervous system (CNS) produces depolarization of those cells. Substance P and acetylcholine have also been shown to have excitatory functions in many regions of the CNS. Examples include the primary afferent terminals of somatosensory fibers within the spinal cord (substance P) and the neuromuscular junction (acetylcholine). Leucine is not known to have transmitter functions.

145. The answer is B. (Kandel, 3rd Ed., pp. 217-221; Cooper, 6th Ed., pp. 382-385, 386-389, 394-400) Thyrotropin-releasing hormone (TRH) and gonadotropin-releasing hormone (GnRH) are examples of neuroactive peptides that are synthesized in the hypothalamus and are released into the portal circulation where they are carried to targets in the anterior pituitary gland. They stimulate the release of thyrotropin and leutenizing hormone and/or follicle stimulating hormone, respectively. One of the more interesting features concerning recent research findings with neuroactive peptides is that the gut peptides such as cholycystokinin, somatostatin, bombesin, and substance P are also found widely throughout the brain. Newly developed immunocytochemical methods now permit an investigator to accurately identify and map the locations of different neuroactive peptides such as somatostatin and met- and leu-enkephalin within the central nervous system. As a result of such mapping studies, it has been shown that a number of the neuroactive peptides are colocalized within the same cell body with other transmitters such as the monoamines. It is likely that neuropeptides, in addition to their other functions, serve to modulate the activity and release of the monoamines.

146. The answer is E. (Cooper, 6th Ed., pp. 38, 149-151, 156, 166-167, 401-409) Electrophysiological and pharmacological studies have established that glycine is an inhibitory transmitter within the spinal cord (and perhaps elsewhere) and that gamma-aminobutyric acid (GABA) is an inhibitory transmitter over wide regions of the central nervous system. Other studies have also established that, in general, enkephalins are largely inhibitory, although several exceptions have recently been reported in the literature. While a neurotransmitter role has yet to be firmly estblished, it has been shown that enkephalins inhibit neuronal activity. Strychnine has been used as an antagonist for glycine, which is an inhibitory transmitter. Muscimol is a GABA agonist.

147. The answer is C. (Cooper, 6th Ed., pp. 209-210, 215-216, 324) The systemic administration of either atropine or scopolamine results in a decrease in brain acetylcholine content. Haloperidol is a dopamine receptor blocker. Physostigmine is an anticholinesterase agent that can reverse the central effects of atropine and other antimuscarinic drugs. Hemicholinium has been shown to block the transport mechanism associated with the accumulation of choline in axon terminals. In this manner, it reduces the amount of acetylcholine present in the brain.

148. The answer is A. (Cooper, 6th Ed., pp. 224-227; Kandel, 3rd Ed., p. 993) Phenylketonuria (PKU) is caused by a deficiency (i.e., structural mutation) in phenylalanine hydroxylase which has significantly reduced levels of enzyme activity. This defect results in abnormally high levels of phenylalanine with diminished levels of tyrosine. An accumulation of phenylalanine can result in brain damage whose features include mental retardation, seizures, and aggressive tendencies.

149. The answer is D. (Cooper, 6th Ed., pp. 244-250) Reserpine interferes with the uptake-storage mechanism associated with amine granules, which results in destruction of these granules. Administration of this drug will produce long-lasting depletion of norepinephrine. Amphetamine blocks the reuptake mechanism and thus produces a net increase in the release of norepinephrine. Apomorphine is a nonspecific dopamine agonist, clonidine is an alpha-2 receptor agonist, and yohimbine is an alpha-2 receptor antagonist.

150. The answer is C. (Cooper, 6th Ed., p. 290; Kandel, 3rd Ed., pp. 207-208) These findings can best be explained in terms of a mechanism that involves presynaptic autoreceptors. These receptors modulate the release of a catecholamine by responding to the concentration of this transmitter within the synapse. It thus represents a specific negative feedback mechanism. For example, if the concentration of transmitter in the synapse is high, then release would likely be inhibited. Less inhibition (i.e., more transmitter release) would occur if concentrations are low. Other choices are obviously incorrect. The presence of a GABAergic neuron at the synapse, postsynaptic inhibition, and collateral inhibition are unrelated since they refer to events associated with the postsynaptic neuron, not the catecholamine (presynaptic) neuron. As a result of the phasic nature of this phenomenon, destruction of the catecholamine cell body would produce events that were not phasic; indeed, there would be permanent loss of the neuron's capacity to release transmitter.

151. The answer is A. (Kandel, 3rd Ed., pp. 226-233) Transmitters such as the catecholamines and acetylcholine have been shown to be actively taken up into synaptic vesicles as a result of differences in pH between the vesicle interior and the cytoplasm. Dissociation of a proton leaves a catecholamine molecule uncharged. The amine, which is now neutral, is transported through the membrane by a carrier into the vesicle. Once inside the vesicle, the amine becomes protonated and is trapped there. Synaptic vesicles are transported down the axon from the Golgi apparatus, and after they are used, are returned to the cell body for recycling. Vesicles also contribute to the release of transmitter via an exocytotic process facilitated by specialized endings of membranes present in the active zone. In this process, the movement of the vesicle to the active zone is mediated by parts of the cytoskeleton. The protein caldesmin, a part of the vesicle membrane, binds actin filaments, tubulin, and calcium ions.

152. The answer is E. (Kandel, 3rd Ed., pp. 232-233) There are three mechanisms by which a transmitter is removed from the region of the synaptic cleft. The most common one is reuptake in which transporter molecules mediate high affinity reuptake that is specific for the transmitter in question. Other mechanisms include diffusion, which removes some components of the transmitter substance, and enzymatic degradation of the amine achieved by the enzymes monoamine oxidase and catechol-O- methyltransferase.

153. The answer is B. (Kandel, 3rd Ed., pp. 235-243) Myasthenia gravis is an autoimmune disease that affects acetylcholine receptors in the postsynaptic membrane of the neuromuscular junction. Patients present with weakness and fatigue that becomes exacerbated with exercise. Experimental studies have revealed that there are distinct morphological changes at the neuromuscular junction. In particular, the junctional folds are more sparse and shallow, which, in effect, produces a widening of the synaptic space and results in an increased diffusion of acetylcholine away from the synaptic cleft. The end result is that transmitter has a lowered probability of interacting with receptors. Accordingly, transmission is reduced or blocked, leading to a marked reduction in the size of the end-plate potential as compared with normal. Other data suggest there is a significant reduction in the number of acetylcholine receptors on the postsynaptic membrane. The destruction of postsynaptic receptors appears to be mediated by antibodies directed against them. It appears these antibodies are directed against a segment of the alpha-subunit referred to as the primary immunogenic region. The destruction of postsynaptic receptors is facilitated by cross linking of receptors by antibody. In myasthenic patients, there is often an abnormality of the thymus gland. It is believed that an initial inflammatory response in the thymus may result in the cross reaction of antibodies that ultimately are directed against acetylcholine receptors. For this reason, thymectomies are frequently carried out and have met with partial success.

154. The answer is C. (Kandel, 3rd Ed., pp. 244-256) The motor unit was originally defined by Sherrington as the basic unit involved in motor functions. It consists of a motor neuron and all of the muscle fibers innervated by that neuron. Note that an individual motor neuron may have a number of terminal branches, each of which innervates a different muscle fiber. Thus, a motor unit will comprise a single motor neuron and many individual muscle fibers. Muscle atrophy is a "wasting away" of that muscle. It occurs when the motor neuron that directly innervates a muscle is damaged and no longer provides effective neural input. Upper motor neurons do not directly innervate muscles and, thus, their effects upon muscle function are quite different. To better evaluate clinical disorders involving neuropathies, it is useful to distinguish between fasciculations and fibrillations. Fasciculations result from involuntary, synchronous contractions of muscle fibers that are innervated by the same motor neuron (i.e., a motor unit). In contrast, fibrillations refer to the spontaneous contractions of single muscle fibers. Conduction velocity along a nerve is enhanced considerably by the presence of myelin. Myelin serves to increase the space constant, and, consequently, current is shunted to the next node of Ranvier (i.e., saltatory conduction ensues). If myelin is removed by a disease process, the space constant is reduced, saltatory conduction is reduced or eliminated, and conduction velocities are lowered.

The Spinal Cord

DIRECTIONS: The questions below consist of lettered headings followed by a set of numbered items. For each numbered item select the **one** heading with which it is **most** closely associated. Each lettered heading may be used **once, more than once, or not at all.**

Questions 155-160

(A) amyotrophic lateral sclerosis

(B) hemisection of the spinal cord

(C) multiple sclerosis

(D) neurological manifestations of pernicious anemia involving vitamin B12 deficiency

(E) syringomyelia

(F) tabes dorsalis

(G) Bell's palsy

155. ipsilateral loss of position sense and contralateral loss of pain and temperature, both below the level of the lesion

156. deficit is limited to a 1-2 segmental loss of pain and temperature, bilaterally with additional evidence of an ipsilateral lower motor neuron paralysis and Horner's syndrome

157. bilateral loss of position sense and bilateral upper motor neuron paralysis

158. evidence of bilateral upper and lower motor neuron paralysis

159. loss of position and vibratory sense with accompanying ataxia

160. demyelinating disease affecting the white matter of the brain and spinal cord, which causes a reduced conduction velocity

DIRECTIONS: The questions below consist of lettered headings followed by a set of numbered items. For each numbered item select the **one** heading with which it is **most** closely associated. Each lettered heading may be used **once, more than once, or not at all.**

Questions 161-165

        (A) unmyelinated C-fibers

        (B) extrafusal muscle fibers

        (C) polar region of muscle spindle

        (D) 1A fibers

        (E) general visceral efferent fibers

        (F) high threshold receptor

        (G) ipsilateral flexion and contralateral extension

161. alpha motor neurons

162. gamma motor neurons

163. withdrawal reflex

164. Golgi tendon organ

165. intermediolateral cell column

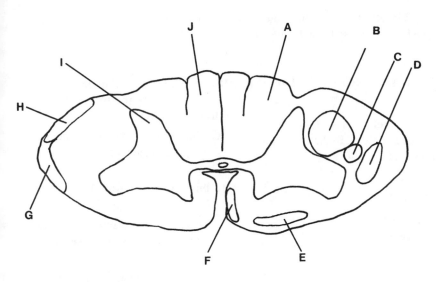

Questions 166-178   Refer to the figure above.

166. second-order neurons that transmit information from muscle spindles to cerebellum

167. first-order neurons that transmit sensory information from the upper limbs to the medulla

168. transmits sensory information directly to the thalamus

169. these fibers originate from the contralateral cerebral cortex

170. this region of spinal cord receives direct sensory inputs from pain and temperature fibers

171. these fibers reach the cerebellum via the superior cerebellar peduncle

172. these fibers facilitate extensor motor neurons

173. these fibers originate in the midbrain and are associated with regulation of flexor motor neurons

174. these fibers originate from the cerebral cortex of the ipsilateral side

175. these fibers mediate joint capsule information from the lower limb

176. destruction of these fibers results in loss of voluntary movements

177. these fibers cross in the lower medulla

178. a surgical lesion of these fibers will alleviate pain from the lower limb

DIRECTIONS: Each question below contains five suggested responses. Select the **one best** response to each question.

Question 179   Refer to the figure on page 53.

179. The level of the section of the spinal cord depicted in the figure on the previous page is:

(A) sacral

(B) lower lumbar

(C) upper lumbar

(D) thoracic

(E) cervical

180. First-order sensory neurons that terminate in laminas I and II of the spinal cord convey mainly:

(A) tactile sensation

(B) pain and temperature sensation

(C) unconscious proprioception limited to inputs from muscle spindles

(D) unconscious proprioception limited to inputs from Golgi tendon organs

(E) inputs associated with pressure receptors

181. It has been established that the transmitter released by the axon terminals of first-order pain and temperature fibers is most likely:

(A) enkephalins

(B) acetylcholine

(C) substance P

(D) gamma aminobutyric acid (GABA)

(E) serotonin

182. Which of the following statements concerning the zone of Lissauer is true :

(A) many fibers that convey unconscious proprioception enter this zone

(B) this zone is composed of coarse, heavily myelinated fibers

(C) fibers within the zone of Lissauer may ascend or descend several segments

(D) these fibers synapse with alpha motor neurons of extensor muscles

(E) cells in this zone typically project to thalamic nuclei

183. Which of the following statements concerning the nucleus dorsalis of Clarke is correct:

(A) it is generally regarded as a nucleus associated with autonomic functions

(B) it contains second-order neurons for the transmission of unconscious proprioceptive information

(C) it contains second-order neurons for the transmission of information from pain receptors

(D) fibers originating from this nucleus cross in the spinal cord

(E) this nucleus is found principally at cervical levels of the cord

184. Which of the following arrange-
ments best describes the somatotopic
organization of the neurons situated in
the ventral horn of the spinal cord:

(A) neurons innervating flexor
muscles lie ventral to those
innervating extensors and neurons
innervating the muscles of the
hand lie lateral to those innervating the trunk

(B) neurons innervating flexor
muscles lie dorsal to those
innervating extensors and neurons
innervating the muscles of the
hand lie medial to those innervating the trunk

(C) neurons innervating flexor
muscles lie dorsal to those
innervating extensors and neurons
innervating the muscles of the
hand lie lateral to those innervating the trunk

(D) neurons innervating the muscles
of the hand lie lateral to those
innervating the trunk but those
innervating flexor and extensor
muscles are not topographically
segregated

(E) neurons innervating the muscles of
the hand lie dorsal to those
innervating the trunk and those
innervating flexor muscles lie
medial to those innervating
extensors

185. All of the following statements
concerning the dorsal columns are true
EXCEPT:

(A) they contain first-order neurons
which synapse in contralateral
dorsal column nuclei

(B) they contain first-order neurons
mediating conscious proprioception from the limbs

(C) sensation from the lower limb is
contained in the fasciculus gracilis
while sensation from the upper
limb is contained in the fasciculus
cuneatus

(D) a lesion of the fasciculus gracilis
may result in ataxia

(E) they contain fibers mediating
either tactile or kinesthetic
sensations, but not both

186. Which of the following pathways all cross in the spinal cord:

(A) lateral spinothalamic tract,
anterior spinothalamic tract,
posterior spinocerebellar tract

(B) anterior spinothalamic tract, lateral
spinothalamic tract, anterior
corticospinal tract

(C) anterior spinocerebellar tract,
posterior spinocerebellar tract,
lateral vestibulospinal tract

(D) anterior corticospinal tract, lateral
spinothalamic tract, dorsal
columns

(E) medial vestibulospinal tract, lateral
spinothalamic tract, anterior
spinothalamic tract

187. All of the following statements concerning the lateral spinothalamic tract are correct EXCEPT:

(A) cells that comprise the origin of the lateral spinothalamic tract arise mainly from laminae IV and V and to a lesser extent from lamina I

(B) cells of this tract cross in the anterior white commissure near their segment of entry

(C) fibers of this tract are somatotopically organized

(D) pain and temperature fibers are anatomically segregated within this tract

(E) lateral spinothalamic fibers terminate exclusively within thalamic nuclei such as VPL, intralaminar nuclei, and posterior thalamic nuclei

188. All of the following statements concerning the cuneocerebellar tract are true EXCEPT:

(A) first-order neurons ascend with the dorsal columns

(B) the accessory cuneate nucleus of the lower medulla constitutes the origin of this pathway

(C) this system of fibers constitutes an ipsilaterally directed pathway from the spinal cord and lower brainstem to the cerebellum

(D) fibers of this tract mediate unconscious proprioception from the lower limb to the cerebellum

(E) the receptors required to activate this system of fibers include muscle spindles and Golgi tendon organs

189. The posterior spinocerebellar and anterior spinocerebellar tracts differ in which of the following ways:

(A) fibers from the posterior spinocerebellar tract enter the cerebellum via the superior cerebellar peduncle, while those from the anterior spinocerebellar tract enter the cerebellum via the inferior cerebellar peduncle

(B) fibers of the posterior spinocerebellar tract mediate impulses from the Golgi tendon organs, while those of the anterior spinocerebellar tract mediate impulses arising from the muscle spindles

(C) fibers associated with the posterior spinocerebellar tract signal whole limb movement, while those associated with the anterior spinocerebellar tract signal information concerning the activity of individual muscles

(D) fibers of the posterior spinocerebellar tract arise from all levels of the spinal cord while those of the anterior spinocerebellar tract arise only from cervical levels

(E) the posterior spinocerebellar tract arises mainly from thoracic levels, while the anterior spinocerebellar tract arises mainly from lumbar levels

190. All of the following statements concerning the corticospinal tract are correct EXCEPT:

(A) fibers of this tract arise from precentral gyrus, postcentral gyrus, and premotor area

(B) fibers of this tract are distributed to all levels of the spinal cord

(C) approximately 80% of corticospinal fibers cross in the pyramidal decussation

(D) the fibers contained in the corticospinal tract are topographically organized in that axons arising from the precentral gyrus synapse upon cells in the dorsal horn while those arising from the postcentral gyrus terminate upon neurons in the ventral horn

(E) lesions of the corticospinal tract produce an upper motor neuron paralysis

191. All of the following concerning a lesion of the pyramidal system are most commonly true EXCEPT:

(A) loss of volitional movement of the limb(s) contralateral to the lesion

(B) spasticity

(C) hypotonia of the limb(s) ipsilateral to the lesion

(D) a positive Babinski sign

(E) a reduction in the size of the internal capsule on the side ipsilateral to the lesion

192. All of the following concerning the rubrospinal tract are true EXCEPT:

(A) the fibers of this tract cross in the brainstem

(B) fibers of this tract arise somatotopically from the red nucleus

(C) fibers of this tract supply both cervical and lumbar levels of the spinal cord

(D) the fibers end directly on ventral horn cells

(E) activation of the red nucleus results in facilitation of flexor motor neurons on the contralateral side of the cord

193. Characteristics of the lateral vestibulospinal tract include all of the following EXCEPT:

(A) arises exclusively from the lateral vestibular nucleus

(B) is somatotopically organized

(C) supplies all levels of the ipsilateral spinal cord

(D) powerfully facilitates alpha motor neurons that innervate extensor muscles

(E) is excited by Purkinje cells of the cerebellum

194. All of the following statements concerning reticulospinal tracts are true EXCEPT:

(A) reticulospinal tracts can modulate cortically induced reflex activity but have little effect on muscle tone

(B) the lateral reticulospinal tract arises from the medial two-thirds of the medullary reticular formation and descends, for the most part, ipsilaterally, to all levels of the cord

(C) the effect of stimulation of cells which give rise to the lateral reticulospinal tract is to suppress movement-related processes

(D) the medial reticulospinal tract arises from the medial aspect of the pontine tegmentum and descends, mainly ipsilaterally, to all levels of the cord and serves to facilitate spinal reflex activity

(E) one component of the descending fibers from the reticular formation contains serotonergic fibers from the nucleus raphe magnus that terminate in the dorsal horn and which likely serve to inhibit sensory neurons in this region

195. Which of the following statements correctly characterizes the descending component of the medial longitudinal fasciculus (MLF):

(A) The descending component of the MLF contains fibers arising from the inferior and lateral vestibular nuclei

(B) The descending component of the MLF contains fibers originating in large part from the medial vestibular nucleus which play a role in the regulation of labyrinthine modulation of head position

(C) Descending fibers of the MLF are contained within the ventrolateral aspect of the white matter of the spinal cord in a position just lateral to the lateral vestibulospinal and lateral reticulospinal tracts

(D) Descending fibers of the MLF suppress extensor reflex activity of the lower limbs of the contralateral side

(E) The descending component of the MLF relays impulses from several forebrain nuclei to the intermediolateral cell column of the spinal cord for the regulation of blood pressure

The Spinal Cord 59

196. An injury to a patient results in a hemisection of the right half of the spinal cord which extends from T8 to T12. It is probable that the patient will experience:

(A) loss of pain and temperature sensation from the right leg; loss of conscious proprioception from the left leg; upper motor neuron paralysis of the left leg

(B) loss of pain and temperature sensation from the left leg; loss of conscious proprioception from the right leg; upper motor neuron paralysis of the left leg

(C) loss of pain and temperature sensation from the left arm and leg; loss of conscious proprioception from the right leg and arm; flaccid paralysis of the right leg

(D) loss of pain and temperature sensation from the left leg and loss of conscious proprioception from the right leg; upper motor neuron paralysis of the right leg

(E) bilateral loss of pain and temperature sensation and conscious proprioception, both from the lower half of the body; upper motor neuron paralysis of the left leg and flaccid paralyis of the right leg

197. All of the following mechanisms or events make it likely that the duration of the stretch reflex will be relatively short EXCEPT:

(A) the action of Renshaw cells

(B) unloading of the spindle by muscle contraction

(C) activation of the Golgi tendon organ

(D) the action of certain cutaneous and joint afferent fibers

(E) activation of gamma motor neurons

198. Which of the following statements concerning muscle spindles is true:

(A) They detect the rate of change of muscle length.

(B) They are high threshold receptors.

(C) They are arranged in series with the extrafusal muscle fibers.

(D) They contain a single type of intrafusal fiber.

(E) They are primarily tension detectors.

199. All of the following statements concerning the stretch reflex are true EXCEPT:

(A) Impulses from dynamic gamma motor neurons that activate dynamic nuclear bag fibers enhance stretch of the central sensory region of the muscle spindle together with the dynamic sensitivity of the primary ending.

(B) The contractile regions of nuclear chain and static bag fibers shorten when stimulated by gamma static efferents, leading to an increase in the steady-state discharge of primary endings.

(C) The stretch reflex consists of two components: a brisk, phasic contraction and a longer lasting tonic contraction.

(D) Golgi tendon organs are basically sensitive to the stretching of a muscle.

(E) One way to determine whether or not a descending fiber bundle from the brainstem modulates motor functions by selective activation of the gamma system would be to stimulate that descending fiber bundle prior to and after cutting the dorsal roots of those fibers associated with the muscle group in question.

200. All of the following statements concerning the muscle action potential and muscle contraction are correct EXCEPT:

(A) The transmitter at the neuromuscular junction is acetylcholine.

(B) The muscle action potential results when transmitter–induced opening of channels allows sodium ions to reach the interior of the muscle fiber membrane at the nerve terminal.

(C) The ultimate effect of a nerve action potential when it reaches the neuromuscular junction is to generate an end-plate potential, which then triggers the muscle action potential.

(D) Inhibition of the muscle action potential can result from inhibitory impulses that reach the neuromuscular junction which serve to close sodium channels.

(E) The contractile process is initiated by the sudden increase in intracellular calcium (from the sarcoplasmic reticulum) which initiates attractive forces between actin and myosin filaments.

201. All of the following statements concerning muscle contractions are correct EXCEPT:

(A) Calcium ions are removed from the intracellular compartment by passive diffusion.

(B) An essential feature of the muscle fiber which enables the contraction to spread throughout the entire fiber is the T-tubule system.

(C) When the T-tubule system is depolarized, specialized channels allow calcium ions to be released throughout the sarcoplasmic reticulum.

(D) Myosin and actin can interact to produce a muscle contraction because calcium ions bind to troponin C.

(E) The force of contraction is a function of the initial length of the muscle

The Spinal Cord

Answers

155-160. The answers are: 155-B, 156-E, 157-D, 158-A, 159-F, 160-C. (Carpenter and Sutin, 8th Ed., pp. 303-314) One of the most striking features of a hemisection of the spinal cord (i.e., Brown-Séquard's syndrome) (B) is the dissociation of loss of pain/temperature with conscious proprioception. On the side ipsilateral to the lesion, there is loss of conscious proprioception since the first-order dorsal column fibers ascend ipsilaterally. In contrast, there is no loss of pain and temperature, ipsilaterally, below the level of the lesion because second-order neurons decussate near their levels of origin and ascend on the contralateral side uninterrupted by the lesion. And, since the pain and temperature fibers, decussate, the second-order ascending fibers conveying information from the contralateral side of the body will be disrupted by the lesion. Fibers associated with conscious proprioception on the contralateral side will be left intact since they remain on the side of entry into the cord. In syringomyelia (E), a development of long cavities in relationship to the central canal frequently extends into the anterior gray horn and region of the intermediolateral cell column. Thus, such a lesion will result in a segmental loss of pain and temperature, bilaterally, and may also cause some additional disruption of autonomic functions. One of these includes Horner's syndrome (i.e., ipsilateral constriction of the pupil, dropping of the upper eyelid, vasodilation, and dryness of the skin of the face) which results from damage to the cell bodies of preganglionic sympathetic neurons. In addition, this lesion extends to the anterior horn where it disrupts lower motor neurons, producing a lower motor neuron or flaccid paralysis of the ipsilateral limb. In combined systems disease (D), there is damage to the dorsal columns with loss of conscious proprioception combined with damage to the corticospinal tracts, which produces an upper motor neuron paralysis. It is caused by a vitamin B12 deficiency. Amyotrophic lateral sclerosis (A) is a degenerative disease that destroys both upper motor neurons (i.e., corticospinal tracts) and lower motor neurons (i.e., ventral horn cells). Thus, this disorder produces signs of both upper and lower motor neuron disturbances. In tabes dorsalis (F), a CNS form of syphilis, degeneration of the central processes of dorsal root ganglion cells ensues, resulting in demyelination of portions of the dorsal columns. This damage results in loss of position and vibration sensations as well as ataxia because of the loss of position sense. In multiple sclerosis (C), demyelination of the white matter of the brain and spinal cord leads to a reduction of conduction velocities, which ultimately produces loss of basic functions that require intact neural circuits.

161-165. The answers are: 161-B, 162-C, 163-G, 164-F, 165-E. (Kandel, 3rd Ed., pp. 569-575, 577, 585-590) Alpha motor neurons innervate extrafusal muscle fibers (B) to produce contraction of the muscle and movement of the limb. Gamma motor neurons innervate the polar region of the muscle spindle(C). When activated, these neurons help to reset the position of the muscle spindle and to increase the likelihood that some external stimulus will activate the spindle. The withdrawal reflex differs from the stretch reflex in that it involves the activation of ipsilateral flexor and contralateral extensor muscles (G). Golgi tendon organs are high-threshold receptors (F) that become activated by whole-limb movement. The intermediolateral cell column of thoracic, lumbar, and sacral levels contains the cell bodies of preganglionic neurons of the sympathetic and parasympathetic nervous systems, respectively. Accordingly, these fibers are classified as general visceral efferent fibers (GVE) (E).

Questions 166-178. The answers are: 166-H, 167-A, 168-D, 169-B, 170-I, 171-G, 172-E, 173-C, 174-F, 175-J, 176-B, 177-B, 178-D. (Carpenter and Sutin, 8th Ed., pp. 265-314) The posterior spinocerebellar tract (H) transmits information from muscle spindles to the cerebellum via the inferior cerebellar peduncle. This tract is located on the lateral aspect of the lateral funiculus of the cord, just above the ventral (anterior) spinocerebellar tract. The ventral spinocerebellar tract supplies the cerebellum via the superior cerebellar peduncle. The sensory fibers that terminate in the medulla are located only in the dorsal columns. The fibers mediating conscious proprioception associated with the upper limbs are contained in the fasciculus cuneatus (A) while those associated with the lower limbs are contained in the fasciculus gracilis (J). The lateral spinothalamic tract (D) transmits pain and temperature information directly to the thalamus. The lateral corticospinal tract (B) originates in the contralateral cortex and crosses over at the level of the lower medulla. This important pathway mediates volitional movements. When these fibers are damaged, there is a clear-cut loss of ability to produce voluntary movement. Surgical destruction of the lateral spinothalamic tract (D) has some-times been used to relieve pain. Pain and temperature fibers from the periphery terminate directly in the region of the dorsal horn called the substantia gelatinosa (I). The lateral vestibulospinal tract (E) powerfully facilitates alpha motor neurons of extensor muscles. The rubrospinal tract (C), situated adjacent to the lateral cortico-spinal tract, originates from the red nucleus of the midbrain and facilitates flexor motor neurons. A smaller component of the corticospinal tract — the anterior corticospinal tract (F) — originates from the cerebral cortex and passes ipsilaterally to the spinal cord. In its position seen in this illustration, the fibers are ipsilateral to their cortical original. Just prior to their termination, many are then distributed to the contralateral side of the cord.

179. The answer is E. (Carpenter and Sutin, 8th Ed., pp. 232-255) The cervical level of the spinal cord can be distinguished from other levels of the cord by the following characteristics: the presence of a well-defined funiculus cuneatus situated immediately lateral to the funiculus gracilis, the presence of well-defined motor nuclei that are clumped into six different groups, three of which can be distinguished, an absence of an intermediolateral cell column, and by its general size — relatively extensive quantities of both white and gray matter.

180. The answer is B. (Carpenter and Sutin, 8th Ed., pp. 243-264) First-order neurons conveying pain and temperature sensations to the spinal cord terminate principally in laminae I and II upon dendrites of cells located in other laminae. For the most part, tactile and pressure sensations are carried by the dorsal column-medial lemniscal systems which terminate in the lower medulla. Fibers mediating unconscious proprioception terminate in the nucleus dorsalis of Clarke.

181. The answer is C. (Carpenter and Sutin, 8th Ed., pp. 246-247, 260-263) Immunocytochemical studies have demonstrated that the terminals of sensory neurons that terminate in laminae I and II of the dorsal horn of the spinal cord stain intensely for substance P. These neurons are believed to mediate pain impulses. Other transmitter substances, while present within the spinal cord, have not been associated directly with first-order sensory afferent fibers.

182. The answer is C. (Carpenter and Sutin, 8th Ed., pp. 257-258) The zone of Lissauer, located on the dorsolateral margin of the dorsal horn of the spinal cord, receives many incoming fibers that are either unmyelinated or finely myelinated. These fibers principally mediate pain and temperature sensations. The fibers contained in this bundle may ascend or descend several segments serving to integrate different levels of the substantia gelatinosa, which receives these inputs. These fibers are not known to make synaptic contact with motor neurons. Neurons in the substantia gelatinosa do not generally ascend beyond the spinal cord.

183. The answer is B. (Carpenter and Sutin, 8th Ed., pp. 250, 256, 276-277) The nucleus dorsalis of Clarke is situated in the medial aspect of lamina VII of the cord at thoracic and lumbar levels, but does extend up to C8. It receives first-order inputs from fibers conveying muscle spindle and Golgi tendon organ information. Fibers from the nucleus dorsalis run laterally to form the dorsal spinocerebellar tract on the ipsilateral side, which terminates mainly in the anterior lobe of the cerebellum.

184. The answer is C. (Carpenter and Sutin, 8th Ed., p. 254) The neurons situated in the ventral horn of the gray matter of the cord are somatotopically organized. This relationship is most clearly seen at cervical levels of the cord. The neurons innervating flexors lie dorsal to those innervating extensors, and the neurons innervating the muscles of the trunk are situated medial to those innervating the hand. These relationships take on added significance when one considers the nature of the descending motor pathways that synapse with these cells. For example, fibers associated mainly with the control of the flexor musculature, such as the corticospinal and rubrospinal tracts, are situated at relatively dorsal levels of the lateral funiculus of the cord. Similarly, fibers associated with the regulation of antigravity muscles (i.e., generally the extensor musculature) are situated in a more ventral position. Thus, the somatotopic organization is maintained throughout the brain stem as well as the spinal cord.

185. The answer is A. (Carpenter and Sutin, 8th Ed., pp. 265-270) The dorsal column system is a highly discriminating system in which a given fiber pathway is generally responsive to a single modality of sensory input. It contains first-order neurons that ascend ipsilaterally to the lower medulla where they synapse with corresponding dorsal column nuclei. Conscious proprioception from the lower limbs is mediated via the fasciculus gracilis, while the same modality of sensation from the upper limb is mediated via the fasciculus cuneatus. A lesion of the fasciculus gracilis will result in the loss of conscious awareness of one's position sense. Accordingly, it could likely result in the development of ataxic movements, which is defined as an error in the range, force, and direction of movement.

186. The answer is B. (Carpenter and Sutin, 8th Ed., pp. 265-306) Both the lateral and anterior spinothalamic tracts cross over to the contralateral white matter of the cord relatively close to their cell bodies of origin and ascend to the thalamus. Similarly, the ventral spinocerebellar tract crosses over to the contralateral side and ascends as a distinct fiber pathway in the far lateral aspect of the white matter immediately below the position occupied by the dorsal spinocerebellar tract. The anterior corticospinal tract represents approximately 10% of the fibers descending from the cortex as corticospinal fibers. These fibers pass ipsilaterally through the brainstem to the spinal cord, reaching the anterior funiculus of the cord. Near the level at which these fibers terminate, most anterior corticospinal fibers cross over in the commissure of the spinal cord to supply the intermediate gray of the ventral horn. Posterior spinocerebellar fibers, which arise from the nucleus dorsalis of Clarke, do not cross in the spinal cord. Instead, they pass laterally from their cell of origin and ascend within the dorsal half of the far lateral aspect of the white matter to the cerebellum. Lateral vestibulospinal fibers arise from the lateral vestibular nucleus and descend ipsilaterally within the ventral funiculus to all levels of the spinal cord where they terminate upon neurons in the ventral horn. Dorsal column fibers are first-order neurons that arise from the periphery and enter the spinal cord at all levels. They ascend ipsilaterally in the dorsal columns to the level of the dorsal column nuclei of the medulla where they terminate.

187. The answer is E. (Carpenter and Sutin, 8th Ed., pp. 270-274) Fibers of the lateral spinothalamic tract arise mainly from laminae IV, V, and I (to a small extent). The fibers cross in the anterior white commissure near their level of origin, ascend in a somatotopic manner (in which pain and temperature fibers are segregated) as the lateral spinothalamic tract to terminate in several nuclear groups of the thalamus. In addition, many collaterals of the spinothalamic fibers also terminate throughout the reticular formation of the medulla and pons.

188. The answer is D. (Carpenter and Sutin, 8th Ed., pp. 276-280) The cuneocerebellar and dorsal spinocerebellar tracts are functionally similar. However, the latter conveys information from muscle spindles and Golgi tendon organs to the cerebellum from the upper limb, while the former conveys similar information to the cerebellum from the lower limb. First-order neurons mediating inputs associated with unconscious proprioception from the upper limb pass directly (and ipsilaterally) through the fasciculus cuneatus to the accessory cuneate nucleus. Second-order neurons from this nucleus then pass laterally as external arcuate fibers which enter the ipsilateral cerebellum via the inferior cerebellar peduncle.

189. The answer is E. (Carpenter and Sutin, 8th Ed., pp. 276-279) The posterior spinocerebellar tract carries impulses from both muscle spindles and Golgi tendon organs to the cerebellum via the inferior cerebellar peduncle. The anterior spinocerebellar tract supplies inputs to the cerebellum via the superior cerebellar peduncle. The two tracts differ anatomically since the posterior spinocerebellar tract arises mainly from thoracic levels (C8-L2 or L3) while the anterior spinocerebellar tract arises mainly from lumbar levels. The inputs from the anterior spinocerebellar tract are from the Golgi tendon organ. Thus, these tracts also differ functionally in that the dorsal spinocerebellar tract signals information associated with individual muscles, while the anterior spinocerebellar tract signals information associated with groups of muscles (i.e., whole limb movements).

190. The correct answer is D. (Carpenter and Sutin, 8th Ed., pp. 282-288) The corticospinal tract arises from the precentral gyrus (area 4, 30%), postcentral gyrus (areas 3,1,2, 40%), and premotor area (area 6, 30%). Distribution of these fibers to all levels of the cord provides the anatomical substrate for voluntary control over somatic and autonomic functions. The majority of fibers (75-90%) arising from the cortex cross in the pyramidal decussation and terminate in the contralateral side of the cord. Thus, a lesion along this tract above the decussation of the pyramids will result in an upper motor neuron paralysis associated with the contralateral side of the body. The fibers from the postcentral gyrus (i.e., primary sensory cortex) make synapse in the dorsal horn of the cord which is associated with incoming sensory signals. In contrast, fibers from the precentral gyrus (i.e., primary motor cortex) synapse in the ventral horn of the cord. In this manner, descending cortical fibers may serve several functions: (1) to activate motor horn cells for the initiation of movement and (2) to regulate incoming sensory information that might otherwise be directed to the parietal lobe.

191. The answer is C. (Carpenter and Sutin, 8th Ed., pp. 282-288) Lesions of the cortex associated with the origin of the corticospinal tracts (such as the motor cortex, postcentral gyrus, and/or premotor area) or along the pathway for this system (e.g., internal capsule) produce a constellation of deficits that are characteristic of lesions of this pathway. These include: paralysis of the contralateral limb(s), hyperreflexia, spasticity, and a positive Babinski sign. Because the cell bodies of origin of this pathway have been damaged, Wallerian degeneration ensues and this reduces the size of the internal capsule through which the corticospinal tract passes. This can be readily observed on a CAT scan of the brain of such a patient. Typically, the limbs on the side ipsilateral to the site of the lesion are unaffected by the lesion.

192. The answer is D. (Carpenter and Sutin, 8th Ed., pp. 290-293) The rubrospinal tract originates from the red nucleus. The pathway is somatotopically organized. Cells situated in more dorsal aspects of this nucleus supply the cervical cord while those situated more ventral supply the lumbar cord. The pathway decussates close to its origin in the ventral tegmentum of the midbrain, thus enabling it to influence spinal neurons of the contralateral cord. The characteristic effect of stimulation of this system is facilitation of flexor motor neurons. This is accomplished not by direct connections from red nucleus to ventral horn cells but through interneurons inasmuch as rubrospinal fibers terminate in intermediate levels of the cord (i.e., laminae VI-VII).

193. The answer is E. (Carpenter and Sutin, 8th Ed., pp. 293-295) The lateral vestibular nucleus gives rise to an important somatotopically organized tract that descends ipsilaterally to all levels of the spinal cord. The cervical cord receives inputs arising from ventro-rostral levels, and the lumbar-sacral cord receives inputs from dorsal-caudal levels of the lateral vestibular nucleus. Activation of the lateral vestibular nucleus results in significant excitation of alpha motor neurons of extensors and corresponding facilitation of extensor reflexes. Purkinje cells of the cerebellum inhibit all neurons with which they synapse, including the lateral vestibular nucleus.

194. The answer is A. (Carpenter and Sutin, 8th Ed., pp. 295-298) One of the most significant features of the reticulospinal fibers is that they can exert powerful modulatory actions on motor processes at the level of the spinal cord. Such effects may occur through modulation of alpha or gamma motor neurons, resulting in the regulation of cortically induced reflex activity or reflex activity initiated at spinal levels. In particular, the reticular formation appears to selectively target the gamma motor system in modulating motor activity. Accordingly, such modulation will produce profound effects upon muscle spindle activity and, ultimately, on muscle tone. Stimulation of different parts of the reticular formation produces different effects on spinal reflex activity. The lateral reticulospinal tract, which arises from the medial two-thirds of the medulla, projects to all levels of the cord and generates a suppressive effect. The medial reticulospinal tract, which arises from the pontine tegmentum, facilitates reflex activity. In addition, fibers from the nucleus raphe magnus of the medulla descend to the dorsal horn of the cord where they serve to inhibit incoming sensory impulses that are associated most closely with pain sensations.

195. The answer is B. (Carpenter and Sutin, 8th Ed., p. 298) This pathway originates, in large measure, in the medial vestibular nucleus although other regions such as the interstitial nucleus of Cajal of the midbrain, superior colliculus (by virtue of the tectospinal tract), and reticular formation also contribute fibers to this bundle. Fibers from the inferior vestibular nucleus project, instead, to the cerebellum and contribute a few fibers to the ascending component of the MLF; the lateral vestibular nucleus is the origin of the lateral vestibulospinal tract and this cell group also contributes fibers to the ascending component of the MLF. A principal descending component of the MLF arises from the medial vestibular nucleus, and, accordingly, this bundle is sometimes referred to as the medial vestibulospinal tract. The overall function of the MLF is to help coordinate changes in position or balance with the position of the head and eyes. The descending fibers of the MLF provide the anatomical substrate by which the inputs from the vestibular apparatus can influence the manner in which the head will be positioned. It accomplishes this by modulating upper cervical neurons which innervate muscles of the neck that control the position of the head. Since the projection is to the cervical cord, it would not likely have any direct effect upon extensor reflex activity of the lower limbs. Likewise, these descending fibers do not affect any structures that would cause alterations in blood pressure.

196. The answer is D. (Carpenter and Sutin, 8th Ed., pp. 310-312) Hemisection of the right side of the spinal cord involving segments T8 to T12 will result in contralateral loss of pain and temperature sensation below the level of the lesion and ipsilateral loss of conscious proprioception below the level of the lesion. Thus, this patient will experience loss of pain and temperature in the left leg and loss of conscious proprioception in the right leg. In addition, there will be damage to the descending corticospinal fibers that normally are essential for activation of the lower motor neurons controlling muscles of the right leg (i.e., upper motor neuron paralysis of the right leg). However, since the lesion is situated below the entry of sensory fibers as well as the origin of anterior horn cells that innervate the upper limbs, no loss of sensation to the upper limbs will ensue, nor will there be a lower or upper motor neuron paralysis of the upper limbs. The pain and temperature fibers ipsilateral to the site of the lesion are unaffected because the second-order neurons decussate at the approximate level of their cell bodies of origin and ascend on the side contralateral to the lesion, leaving this system intact.

197. The answer is E. (Kandel, 3rd Ed., pp. 565-586) Alpha motor neurons innervate the extrafusal muscle fibers of muscles. When the alpha motor neuron of an extensor muscle is activated by a 1A sensory afferent as part of the stretch (myotatic) reflex, an axon collateral of the alpha motor neuron also causes an interneuron, called a Renshaw cell, to discharge. The Renshaw cell is an inhibitory interneuron that synapses with this alpha motor neuron. By doing so, it causes the alpha motor neuron to cease firing. Since the reflex is initially activated by impulses in the 1A fibers generated by the muscle spindle when it is stretched (i.e., loaded), further impulses along the 1A pathway cease when the spindle is unloaded (i.e., released from stretch). In this situation, the intrafusal fibers slacken and the firing rate of the afferent endings decrease or terminate. This is sometimes referred to as the silent period of the spindle. The stretch reflex cannot continue because its afferent limb has become inactivated. In addition, the stretch reflex may be terminated by the activation of the Golgi tendon organ. This receptor becomes activated when the extrafusal muscles contract (i.e., limb movement associated with the stretch reflex). As a result, a number of other fiber groups now become activated. The Golgi tendon organ gives rise to a 1B afferent fiber that synapses upon an inhibitory interneuron to the alpha motor neuron governing the stretch reflex. Moreover, this inhibitory interneuron also receives convergent input from muscle spindles associated with neighboring muscle groups, cutaneous afferents, and joint afferents, all of which facilitate its activation. This arrangement ultimately inhibits the extensor motor neuron from discharging again and thus reduces the duration of the stretch reflex. Gamma motor neurons facilitate the discharge of the muscle spindle.

198. The answer is A.   (Kandel, 3rd Ed., pp. 569-579) In contrast to Golgi tendon organs which detect tension, muscle spindles respond to the rate of change in the length of the muscle and are referred to as velocity detectors. They are low threshold detectors and are connected in parallel with the extrafusal muscle fibers. Stretching the muscle results in an elongation of intrafusal fibers, which stretches the sensory nerve endings in the spindle, producing an increase in the discharge rate. The muscle spindle actually contains three different types of intrafusal fibers: dynamic nuclear bag, static nuclear bag, and nuclear chain fibers, all of which are innervated by a single 1A afferent fiber. Static nuclear bag fibers and nuclear chain fibers are innervated by group II afferent fibers. The various properties of these intrafusal fibers combine in generating the firing patterns of the spindle.

199. The answer is D.   (Kandel, 3rd Ed., pp. 566-574, 577-578, 583-586) Because the Golgi tendon organ is in series with the muscle, stretching the muscle does not constitute a sufficient stimulus to activate this receptor. Instead, it acts as a tension receptor, responding to sudden changes in the tension of the muscle generated by either stretching the tendon or by contraction of the muscle. When dynamic nuclear bag fibers are activated by dynamic gamma motor neurons, the polar regions display a viscous response. This effect leads to a lengthening in the central region of the fiber causing an increase in the dynamic sensitivity of the primary ending. In contrast, nuclear chain and bag fibers shorten when stimulated, which results in an increase in the steady-state discharge rate of the primary and secondary endings. The stretch reflex, therefore, consists of two components: a phasic contraction produced by a sudden change in the length of the muscle, and a tonic contraction produced by the (static) adjustment of the muscle to a different length. To determine whether a descending fiber system from the brainstem selectively modulates the gamma motor system, one can simply cut the dorsal roots.

If the effects generated prior to the cut are no longer present after the cut, the conclusion is that gamma efferents are involved in modulation induced from this descending   brainstem pathway. The rationale here is that, by cutting the dorsal roots (which include 1A fibres), the effects of the gamma system have been eliminated because this system can only be functional when 1A fibers are activated. Said otherwise, the gamma loop requires the following circuit: gamma motor neurons —> activation of 1A fibers —> alpha motor neuron activation —> contraction of the extrafusal muscle fiber.

200. The answer is D.   (Kandel, pp. 548-553; Guyton, 2nd Ed., pp. 295-306, 308-311) As a general rule, inhibition of motor functions occurs within the CNS, not in the periphery. The only neural connections of nerve to muscle include the alpha and gamma motor neurons (which are excitatory) and the 1A sensory fibers whose receptor is contained within the intrafusal muscle fiber. When an impulse arrives at the neuromuscular junction from a motor neuron, it releases the transmitter, acetylcholine, into the junction. This results in the opening of acetylcholine-gated ion channels which permit sodium ions to reach the inside of the fiber, creating the local end-plate potential. The local end-plate potential, in turn, triggers a muscle action potential. The sudden release of large quantities of calcium ions into the sarcoplasm adjoining the myofibrils serves to activate forces between the filaments which leads to contraction of the muscle fiber.

201. The answer is A.   (Kandel, 3rd Ed., pp. 549-553; Guyton, 2nd Ed., pp. 297-302) The T-tubules are in communication with the extracellular fluid surrounding the muscle fiber and therefore contain extracellular fluid. Since the action potential spreads over the muscle fiber membrane, it also spreads through the T-tubule system to much of the muscle fiber. An essential feature of the T-tubule system is that its depolarization affects voltage-sensitive channels in the terminal cisternae resulting in the release of calcium ions throughout the sarcoplasmic reticulum. Eventually, calcium is removed from the intracellular space by an active transport system. However, its presence is critical for the interaction of myosin and actin. Calcium ions bind to troponin C, which permits a conformational change in the actin molecule whereby the myosin head is now exposed to a receptor site. The initial length of the muscle is a factor in determining the force of contraction.   The contractile force of a muscle is a function of the degree of overlap between the actin filaments and the cross bridges of the myosin filaments. Thus, the greater the number of cross bridges that pull on the actin filaments, the greater will be the contractile strength.

Autonomic Nervous System

DIRECTIONS: Each question below contains five suggested responses. Select the **one best** response to each question.

202. All of the following statements concerning the parasympathetic nervous system are correct EXCEPT:

(A) The origins of the preganglionic neurons are sacral levels S2-S4 and cranial nerves III, VII, IX and X.

(B) The transmitter released at preganglionic endings is acetylcholine.

(C) The transmitter released at postganglionic endings is norepinephrine.

(D) Preganglionic neurons are regulated by descending fibers from the forebrain.

(E) The cell bodies of postganglionic neurons generally are located close to the organ innervated by their fibers.

203. Effects of sympathetic nervous system activity include all of the following EXCEPT:

(A) pupillary dilation

(B) acceleration of heart rate

(C) dilation of blood vessels of the extremities and the trunk

(D) inhibition of gastric motility

(E) secretion from the adrenal medulla

204. Synaptic transmission in autonomic ganglia is primarily:

(A) cholinergic

(B) noradrenergic

(C) serotonergic

(D) GABAergic

(E) peptidergic

205. Which of the following statements concerning the function of peptides in the autonomic nervous system is true:

(A) They are present only at preganglionic axon terminals of the parasympathetic nervous system.

(B) They are present only at postganglionic axon terminals of the parasympathetic nervous system.

(C) They are present in sympathetic ganglia where they function primarily as neurotransmitters.

(D) They are present in sympathetic ganglia where they function primarily as neuromodulators.

(E) They have not been localized in any of the autonomic ganglia.

206. The carotid sinus reflex involves:

(A) baroreceptor afferent fibers from
the cranial nerve XI

(B) glossopharyngeal efferent fibers

(C) interneurons within the nucleus
ambiguus of the medulla

(D) efferent fibers contained in the
intermediate component of the
facial nerve

(E) vagal efferent fibers

207. Calcium currents present in heart
muscle cells are:

(A) reduced by norepinephrine acting
through beta receptors

(B) increased by norepinephrine
acting through beta receptors

(C) increased by norepinephrine
acting through alpha receptors

(C) increased by acetylcholine acting
on muscarinic receptors

(D) increased by acetylcholine acting
on nicotinic receptors

(E) increased by serotonin acting on
serotonin 1_A receptors

208. All of the following statements
are direct or indirect effects of vagal
stimulation on the heart EXCEPT:

(A) It causes a shortening of the
duration of the action potential.

(B) Cells in the sinoatrial node are
depolarized.

(C) It causes an increase in resting
potassium conductance.

(D) It increases the threshold associated with the pacemaker current.

(E) It acts upon muscarinic receptors.

209. Bladder functions are regulated by
which of the following combinations of
inputs:

(A) vagal and sacral efferent fibers
only

(B) vagal, sacral, and descending
fibers from the cerebral cortex

(C) lumbar and sacral efferent fibers
only

(D) lumbar, sacral, and descending
fibers from the cerebral cortex

(E) lumbar, thoracic, and cervical
fibers only

210. Horner's syndrome can be the
result of damage to all of the following EXCEPT:

(A) descending fibers from the
hypothalamus

(B) postganglionic fibers in the
superior cervical ganglion

(C) preganglionic neurons arising
from the region of the intermediolateral cell column of T1

(D) vagal efferent fibers

(E) fibers in the ventrolateral medulla
which receive hypothalamic
afferents and which project to the
intermediolateral cell column at
thoracic levels of the cord

211. Physiological differences in the effects of norepinephrine and epinephrine released from the adrenal medulla include all of the following EXCEPT:

(A) epinephrine has a more potent effect upon cardiac rate than does norepinephrine

(B) epinephrine is less effective than norepinephrine in constricting blood vessels of skeletal muscles

(C) epinephrine is less effective than norepinephrine in elevating arterial pressure

(D) epinephrine is less effective than norepinephrine in stimulating beta receptor activity

(E) epinephrine has a much more potent effect than norepinephrine upon metabolism

212. A systemic dose of norepinephrine is given and resulting forearm blood flow and blood pressure are measured. The stellate ganglion is removed and 5 weeks later the same dose of norepinephrine is administered. You would expect to observe:

(A) a much greater increase in blood flow in the forearm than prior to the ganglionectomy

(B) a much greater decrease in blood flow in the forearm than prior to the ganglionectomy

(C) no change in blood flow to the forearm

(D) dilation of the blood vessels

(E) reduction of overall blood pressure

213. The hypothalamus and amygdala are able to modulate the output of the autonomic nervous system by virtue of their connections with the:

(A) ventrolateral nucleus of the thalamus

(B) nucleus accumbens

(C) solitary nucleus

(D) red nucleus

(E) ventral horn cells at the level of C8 -- T12 of the spinal cord

214. A stress response includes all of the following EXCEPT:

(A) activation of the hypothalamus

(B) increased concentration of blood glucose

(C) increased blood pressure

(D) increased rates of cellular metabolism

(E) increased secretion by stomach glands

215. Synthesis and storage of norepinephrine can be prevented by:

(A) guanethidine

(B) reserpine

(C) phenoxybenzamine

(D) hexamethonium

(E) metoprolol

Autonomic Nervous System

Answers

202. The answer is C. (Kandel et al., 3rd Ed., pp. 763-771; Carpenter and Sutin, 8th Ed., pp. 210-216; Guyton, 2nd Ed., pp. 275-280). The preganglionic neurons of the parasympathetic nervous system arise from S2-S4 of the spinal cord and from cranial nerves III, VII, IX and X of the brainstem. The transmitter released from the endings of these neurons is acetylcholine. Acetylcholine is also released from most (if not all) endings of the postganglionic neurons as well. Descending inputs from a number of forebrain areas have been shown to modulate (directly or indirectly) functions of the parasympathetic nervous system. Such areas include portions of the hypothalamus and components of the limbic system including the amygdala, septal area, anterior cingulate gyrus, and prefrontal cortex. The cell bodies of postganglionic neurons are generally situated close to the organ they innervate. Thus, postganglionic axons are relatively short in length.

203. The answer is C. (Carpenter and Sutin, 8th Ed., p. 224; Kandel et al., 3rd Ed., pp. 763-769). Activation of the sympathetic nervous system results in pupillary dilatation because postganglionic sympathetic neurons innervate pupillary dilator muscles. Heart rate is increased as a result of transmitter release (norepinephrine) from postganglionic endings. Alpha adrenergic innervation of vascular smooth muscle produces vasoconstriction.

204. The answer is A. (Kandel et al., 3rd Ed., pp. 765-767). The transmitter released from preganglionic endings of both sympathetic and parasympathetic fibers is acetylcholine. The other transmitters listed are not involved at this synapse. Evidence in support of this view is derived, in part, from studies that demonstrated that drugs that block nicotinic receptors (e.g., hexamethonium, curare) also block the output of these systems.

205. The answer is D. (Kandel et al., 3rd Ed., pp. 768-772). Recent studies demonstrate that a wide variety of peptides are found within most sympathetic ganglia. Evidence further suggests that these peptides do not act as transmitters, but instead, serve as neuromodulators. In this manner, the action of peptides in autonomic ganglia is to alter the efficiency of neuronal excitability and the effectiveness of cholinergic transmission at autonomic synapses.

206. The answer is E. (Kandel et al., 3rd Ed., pp. 770-772). The carotid sinus reflex involves several neuronal elements. The afferent side of the reflex begins with stretch receptors in the walls of the carotid sinus, These receptors signal "pressure" as a result of stretch of the low capacitance vessel. This causes an afferent volley of action potentials to pass along the glossopharyngeal nerve into the medulla where the fibers synapse with neurons in the solitary nucleus. These neurons, in turn, synapse upon neurons in the dorsal motor nucleus of the vagus nerve whose axons innervate the heart. Activation of this reflex results in a decrease in heart rate and force of contraction. As a consequence of the decrease in cardiac output, there is an ensuing decrease in blood pressure as well.

207. The answer is B. (Kandel et al., 3rd Ed., pp. 770-772). The calcium current of heart muscle cells is enhanced by the release of norepinephrine that acts on beta adrenergic receptors. This effect is additionally mediated by the modulation of potassium current that serves to keep the action potential of the muscle cells constant. The pacemaker current is also affected by this process since its threshold is decreased as a result of activation of beta receptors (which further involves the second messenger system — cAMP dependent protein kinase). Lowering the threshold of the pacemaker current serves to increase heart rate. Serotonin is not involved in postsynaptic regulation of the heart. Acetylcholine has an inhibitory effect upon heart muscle by acting through different mechanisms.

208. The answer is B. (Kandel et al., 3rd Ed., pp. 772-773). Stimulation of the vagus results in a reduction in heart rate. It does so by involving several mechanisms. Acetylcholine released from axon terminals of the vagus acts upon muscarinic receptors causing an increase in potassium conductance. This leads to a hyperpolarization of cells in the sinoatrial node resulting in a slowing of conduction into the A-V node and, therefore, a decrease in heart rate. Acetylcholine causes a shift in the pacemaker current opposite to that observed for norepinephrine, perhaps by decreasing calcium current and/or reducing the synthesis of cAMP. Moreover, the increase in potassium conductance leads to a shortening of the duration of the action potential.

209. The answer is D. (Kandel et al., 3rd Ed., pp. 773-775). The smooth muscle of the bladder is innervated by postganglionic fibers of the sympathetic nervous system that arise from the inferior mesenteric ganglion. This ganglion, in turn, receives its inputs from T12 — L2 of the intermediolateral cell column of the spinal cord. The smooth muscle of the bladder also receives inputs from postganglionic parasympathetic fibers that are innervated by preganglionic fibers arising from S2 — S4. The external sphincter of the bladder (striated muscle) is innervated by ventral horn cells from the spinal cord. These ventral horn cells, in turn, receive inputs from supraspinal neurons that arise, in part, from the cerebral cortex. It is these neurons that form a part of the substrate for voluntary control over bladder functions.

210. The answer is D. (Carpenter and Sutin, 8th Ed., pp. 226-230). Horner's syndrome is characterized by the following symptoms: (1) a constricted eye (smaller pupil than on the opposite side), a drooping eyelid, and dilation of the blood vessels coupled with dryness of the face (absence of sweating) all on the side ipsilateral to the lesion. It results from a lesion of either the central or peripheral components of the pathways associated with activation of the sympathetic nervous system. Descending hypothalamic fibers play a significant role. Similarly, fibers from the ventrolateral medulla constitute an important descending link to the spinal cord from higher regions of the brain. Peripheral components include both preganglionic neurons arising from T1 of the intermediolateral cell column and postganglionic neurons in the superior cervical ganglion which receive inputs from these preganglionic sympathetic fibers. Postganglionic fibers that would be affected include those which innervate pupillary dilator muscles, smooth muscle of the eyelid, and blood vessels of the face and head. In contrast, vagal efferents are associated with parasympathetic functions which are not involved in this syndrome.

211. The answer is D. (Guyton, 2nd Ed., pp. 277-282). It is now reasonably well established that the primary action of norepinephrine is excitation of alpha adrenergic receptors (although beta receptors may also be affected to a slight extent). Epinephrine excites both alpha and beta adrenergic receptors equally. For this reason, heart rate, which is affected principally via beta adrenergic receptors, is influenced by epinephrine to a greater extent than by norepinephrine. In contrast, norepinephrine causes a much greater constriction of blood vessels of muscles than does epinephrine because of the preponderance of alpha adrenergic receptors at the level of the arterioles. Because peripheral vasoconstriction results in elevation of blood pressure, norepinephrine, through alpha adrenergic stimulation, is a more effective pressor agent than is epinephrine. However, epinephrine generates more potent increases in metabolism because it stimulates intracellular adenylate cyclase via beta receptors.

212. The answer is B. (Guyton, 2nd Ed., pp. 280-281). Under normal conditions, administration of norepinephrine will cause a small reduction in blood flow as a result of vasoconstriction. However, when the stellate ganglion is removed, this effect becomes greatly amplified. This is likely due to a "denervation supersensitivity" at the level of the receptors in the muscles that normally receive inputs from postganglionic neurons arising from the stellate ganglion. Although the precise mechanism is not understood, it is likely there is an increase in the density (number) of receptors present in the muscle in response to the reduced number of impulses it receives from the postganglionic fibers. The process by which new receptor proteins are incorporated into cellular membranes requires days or weeks to occur, thus accounting for the fact that the supersensitivity reaction cannot be demonstrated until several weeks after ganglionectomy. As a result of vasoconstriction following administration of norepinephrine, there is an associated increase in arterial blood pressure.

213. The answer is C. (Kandel et al., 3rd Ed., pp. 766-767). The solitary nucleus of the medulla plays a significant role in the neural control of autonomic functions because it receives input from several different regions of the brain that regulate such functions. These inputs include fibers that arise from the hypothalamus, central nucleus of amygdala, midbrain periaqueductal gray, and sensory processes (i.e., visceral afferents) of the glossopharyngeal and vagus nerves. These later signal changes in blood pressure and levels of oxygen and carbon dioxide in the blood. The ventrolateral nucleus of the thalamus, red nucleus of the midbrain, and ventral horn cells of the spinal cord are associated with somatomotor rather than autonomic function. The nucleus accumbens is believed to be associated with motivational processes.

214. The answer is E. (Guyton, 2nd Ed., pp. 277-283). The stress response involves a discharge of different components of the sympathetic nervous system, usually in response to a threatening stimulus. This response mobilizes the necessary energy (glucose) and provides increased muscle blood flow to permit the organism to defend itself in an appropriate manner. Specific responses include increases in glucose concentration, blood pressure, and rates of cellular metabolism. These events are orchestrated by neurons situated in the hypothalamus. In contrast, increased secretion of stomach glands is an effect generated by the parasympathetic nervous system and is not active during periods of stress.

215. The answer is B. (Guyton, 2nd Ed., pp. 283-284). Noradrenergic activity can be blocked by a number of mechanisms. Reserpine, for example, prevents the synthesis and storage of norepinephrine in sympathetic nerve terminals. Guanethidine affects noradrenergic transmission by blocking the release of norepinephrine at the sympathetic endings. Competitive alpha receptor blockers include phenoxybenzamine and phentolamine, whereas metoprolol blocks Beta-1 receptors. Since acetylcholine is the transmitter at preganglionic synapses of both the parasympathetic and sympathetic nervous systems. Hexamethonium is an effective ganglionic blocker at these synapses.

The Brainstem
and Cranial Nerves

DIRECTIONS: The questions below consist of lettered headings followed by a set of numbered items. For each numbered item select the **one** heading with which it is **most** closely associated. Each lettered heading may be used **once, more than once, or not at all.**

Questions 216-228

(A) special somatic afferent (SSA)

(B) special visceral afferent (SVA)

(C) general somatic afferent (GSA)

(D) general visceral afferent (GVA)

(E) general visceral efferent (GVE)

(F) special visceral efferent (SVE)

(G) general somatic efferent (GSE)

216. mesencephalic nucleus of cranial nerve V

217. otic ganglion

218. nodose ganglion

219. pterygopalatine ganglion

220. geniculate ganglion

221. spiral ganglion

222. Scarpa's (vestibular) ganglion

223. superior salivatory nucleus

224. motor nucleus of cranial nerve V

225. Edinger-Westphal nucleus of cranial nerve III

226. superior vestibular nucleus

227. optic nerve

228. ciliary ganglion

Questions 229-244

(A) solitary nucleus

(B) dorsal motor nucleus of cranial
nerve X

(C) inferior salivatory nucleus

(D) carotid sinus

(E) nucleus ambiguus

(F) nucleus cuneatus

(G) dentate nucleus

(H) spinal tract of cranial nerve V

(I) inferior olivary nucleus

(J) medial vestibular nucleus

(K) lateral vestibular nucleus

(L) superior salivatory nucleus

(M) external cuneate nucleus

(N) superior ganglion

(O) inferior ganglion

(P) otic ganglion

229. origin of glossopharyngeal fibers
that innervate pharyngeal muscles

230. origin of preganglionic parasympathetics that innervate the otic
ganglion

231. lesion of this structure eliminates
facial pain

232. origin of fibers that innervate the
larynx

233. receives 1st order baroreceptor
afferents

234. origin of descending fibers of the
medial longitudinal fasciculus (MLF)

235. stimulation of this structure
facilitates lower limb extensor motor
neurons

236. site of baroreceptors

237. stimulation of this general
visceral efferent (GVE) nucleus causes
slowing of the heart rate

238. locus of cell bodies of fibers that
innervate the carotid sinus

239. locus of cell bodies of fibers
that innervate the external ear

240. axons of these cells innervate the
parotid gland

241. stimulation of this structure
directly excites Purkinje cells

242. these neurons project to ventral
posteromedial nucleus (VPM) of the
thalamus

243. a nucleus of the cerebellum

244. a second-order neuron associated
with taste impulses

Questions 245-249

       (A) peripheral lesion limited to the left cranial nerve VI

       (B) lesion of the left cranial nerve III

       (C) lesion of the left cranial nerve IV

       (D) lesion of the right medial longitudinal fasciculus

       (E) lesion of the caudal aspect of the dorsomedial pons

245. inability to move right eye to right side together with inability to smile on right side

246. inability to move left eye medially

247. difficulty in walking down a flight of stairs

248. paresis of right ocular adduction and monocular horizontal nystagmus on left upon attempt to gaze to left

249. inability to gaze to the left with the left eye

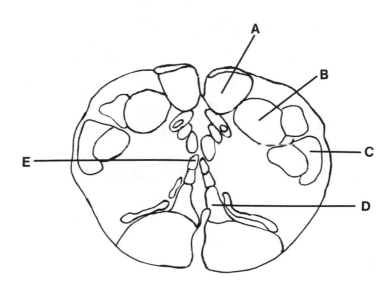

(Adapted from DeArmond, Fig. 41; with permission.)

Questions 250-254 Refer to the figure above.

250. cells in this structure respond to movement of the lower limb

251. cells in this structure respond to a vibratory stimulus applied to the hand

252. fibers in this region mediate reflexes associated with the head

253. first-order pain and temperature fibers

254. these fibers mediate conscious proprioception and 2-point discrimination from the opposite side of the body

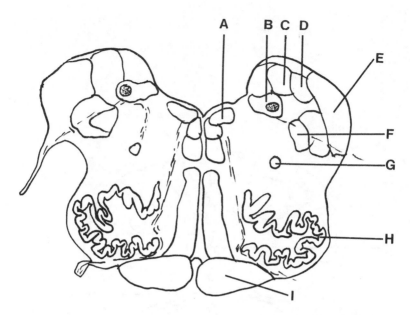

(Adapted from DeArmond, Fig. 44; with permission.)

Questions 255-263   Refer to the figure above.

255. neurons in this structure respond to a taste stimulus

256. neurons in this structure respond to changes in the position of the head and project to the spinal cord

257. neurons here receive inputs from the spinal cord and red nucleus

258. neurons here respond to sudden changes in blood pressure

259. axons of cell in this structure project to the contralateral cerebellar cortex

260. a special visceral efferent (SVE) nucleus

261. a lesion of this structure will produce an upper motor neuron paralysis

262. a general somatic efferent (GSE) nucleus

263. this fiber bundle contains cerebellar afferents arising from the spinal cord and brainstem

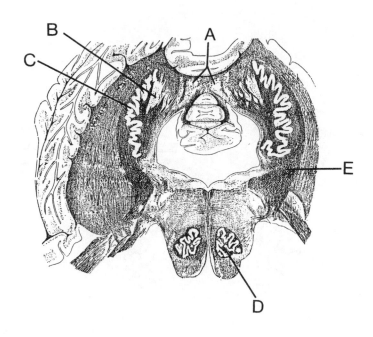

(Adapted from DeArmond, Fig. 14; with permission.)

Questions 264-269   Refer to the figure above.

264. neurons which project to the reticular formation

265. neurons which project to the red nucleus

266. neurons associated with the axial musculature

267. neurons associated with a feedback pathway to the cerebral cortex

268. damage to these neurons is likely to cause nystagmus

269. neurons which project to the ventrolateral (VL) nucleus of the thalamus

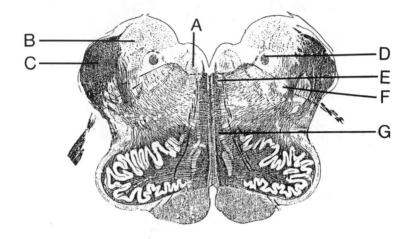

(Adapted from Villiger, Fig. 11; with permission.)

Questions 270-276 Refer to the figure above.

270. receives direct inputs from the vestibular apparatus

271. contains second-order vestibular fibers

272. receives both special visceral afferent and general visceral afferent fibers

273. contains axons which innervate the intrinsic and extrinsic muscles of the tongue

274. fibers which ascend to the thalamus and mediate conscious proprioception

275. mediates pain impulses from the head

276. contains fibers which arise, in part, from the inferior olivary nucleus

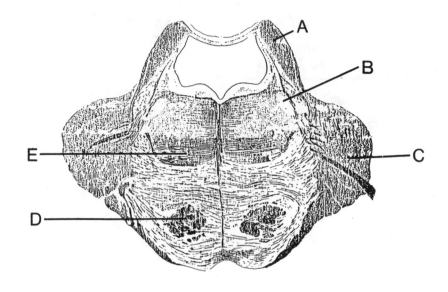

(Adapted from Villiger, Fig. 17; with permission.)

Questions 277-281 Refer to the figure above.

277. axons which are second-order cortico-cerebellar neurons

278. lower motor neurons

279. upper motor neurons

280. these axons which terminate, in part, in the ventrolateral (VL) thalamic nucleus

281. somatotopically organized sensory pathways

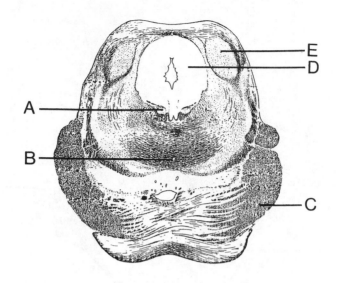

(Adapted from Villiger, Fig. 20; with permission.)

Questions 282-286 Refer to the figure above.

282. sensory relay nucleus

283. fibers which arise from the contralateral dentate and interposed nuclei

284. fibers which arise from the cerebral cortex

285. receives inputs from vestibular structures

286. rich in enkephalin-positive cells and nerve terminals

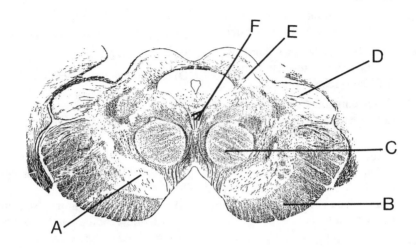

(Adapted from Villiger, Fig. 22; with permission.)

Questions 287-291 Refer to the figure above.

287. neurons in this region respond to moving stimuli

288. specific relay nucleus

289. source of dopaminergic innervation of the striatum

290. receives direct inputs from the cerebellum and cerebral cortex

291. lower motor neurons

DIRECTIONS: Each question below contains five suggested responses. Select the **one best** response to each question.

292. All of the following statements concerning decussation of the pyramids are true EXCEPT:

(A) The decussation is situated in the most caudal part of the medulla.

(B) The fibers contained within this bundle arise exclusively from area 4 of the cerebral cortex.

(C) Fibers contained in this bundle are distributed to all levels of the spinal cord.

(D) Fibers contained in this bundle provide the anatomical substrate by which the left cerebral cortex can mediate voluntary movements of the right limbs.

(E) A complete lesion of the decussation would produce quadriplegia.

293. All of the following statements concerning the dorsal column nuclei are correct EXCEPT:

(A) Collectively, these nuclei are somatotopically organized.

(B) These nuclei display a segregation of sensory modalities.

(C) They receive inputs from first-order neurons associated with sensation in the contralateral limbs.

(D) Axons from dorsal column nuclei form the medial lemniscus.

(E) The principal target nucleus of the dorsal column nuclei is the ventral posterolateral (VPL) nucleus of the thalamus.

294. All of the following tracts are considered first-order sensory pathways EXCEPT:

(A) fasciculus cuneatus

(B) spinal tract of the trigeminal nerve

(C) fasciculus gracilis

(D) external arcuate fibers

(E) fasciculus solitarius

295. Which of the following statements concerning the spinal trigeminal nucleus is correct:

(A) It receives direct inputs from first-order descending sensory fibers contained in the ipsilateral spinal tract of cranial nerve V.

(B) It projects its axons mainly contralaterally to the ventral posterolateral nucleus of the thalamus.

(C) Cells contained in the most caudal aspect of this nucleus respond mainly to mechanical and tactile stimuli.

(D) It receives inputs from primary afferent fibers entering the spinal cord at levels C3 and C4.

(E) It contains cells whose axons project to the hypothalamus.

296. Which of the following features concerning the area postrema is true:

(A) it is located in the ventral medulla at a position caudal to the fourth ventricle

(B) it is considered part of the brain because the cells of this structure are protected by the blood-brain barrier

(C) it plays a role in the regulation of emetic functions

(D) its cells synthesize norepinephrine

(E) it receives major inputs from the forebrain

297. Chemically identified neurons situated within the medulla include all of the following EXCEPT:

(A) norepinephrine

(B) epinephrine

(C) acetylcholine

(D) dopamine

(E) methionine-enkephalin

298. Sources of afferent inputs to the medullary reticular formation include all of the following structures EXCEPT:

(A) the cerebral cortex

(B) collaterals of ascending spinothalamic fibers

(C) the cerebellum

(D) cranial nerve nuclei situated within the medulla

(E) collaterals of dorsal spinocerebellar fibers

299. All of the following statements concerning the inferior olivary complex are correct EXCEPT:

(A) It receives descending inputs from the red nucleus.

(B) Descending inputs come from the cerebral cortex.

(C) It receives direct inputs from ascending spinal fibers.

(D) Fibers arising from the inferior olivary nucleus project to the contralateral cerebellum via the inferior cerebellar peduncle.

(E) Inputs into cerebellum from the inferior olivary nucleus comprise part of the mossy fiber system.

300. All of the following statements about the efferent connections of the medullary reticular formation are correct EXCEPT:

(A) The major descending pathways arise from nuclei situated in the medial two-thirds of the reticular formation.

(B) Fibers arising from the paramedian reticular formation project to the cerebellum.

(C) Cells situated in the lateral third of the reticular formation primarily give rise to long ascending pathways to the forebrain.

(D) Stimulation of the long descending fibers of the medullary reticular formation generally produces inhibition of motor neurons of the spinal cord.

(E) Cells along the midline reticular formation synthesize serotonin and project to the spinal cord.

301. All of the following cranial nerves contain general somatic efferent components (GSE) EXCEPT:

(A) hypoglossal (cranial nerve XII)

(B) trochlear (cranial nerve IV)

(C) trigeminal (cranial nerve V)

(D) occulomotor (cranial nerve III)

(E) abducens (cranial nerve VI)

302. All of the following statements concerning the hypoglossal nerve are true EXCEPT:

(A) Its cell bodies of origin are situated in the dorsomedial aspect of the medulla.

(B) A lower motor neuron lesion involving this nerve will result in deviation of the tongue to the side opposite the lesion.

(C) An upper motor neuron lesion affecting the hypoglossal nerve will also result in deviation of the tongue to the side opposite the lesion.

(D) An upper motor neuron lesion will result in fasciculation of the tongue without producing atrophy of the muscles of the tongue.

(E) A lower motor neuron lesion will produce a flaccid paralysis of the tongue.

303. All of the following statements concerning cranial nerve XI (accessory nerve) are correct EXCEPT:

(A) The cell bodies are located in the lateral aspect of the anterior gray matter of the upper few segments of the cervical cord.

(B) The fibers of this nerve exit via the jugular foramen.

(C) A lesion of this nerve will cause the patient to experience a dropping of the shoulder on the affected side and downward and outward rotation of the scapula.

(D) A lesion of this nerve will also cause a weakness in rotation of the head and an upward tilting of the chin to the opposite side.

(E) This nerve includes a special visceral efferent (SVE) component that innervates the sternomastoid and trapezius muscles and a general somatic afferent (GSA) component that conveys pressure and touch information from the shoulder region.

304. The vagus nerve (cranial nerve X) includes which of the following components:

(A) general somatic afferent, special visceral afferent, general visceral afferent, and general visceral efferent

(B) special visceral afferent, special sensory afferent, general visceral afferent, and general visceral efferent

(C) general visceral afferent and general visceral efferent only

(D) general visceral efferent and special visceral efferent only

(E) special visceral efferent, general visceral efferent, and general visceral afferent only

305. All of the following statements concerning the glossopharyngeal nerve are true EXCEPT:

(A) It is a complex nerve similar to the vagus but does not contain a general visceral efferent (GVE) component.

(B) It receives a general somatic afferent (GSA) input from the external ear.

(C) It receives special visceral afferent (SVA) inputs from the carotid body and posterior third of the tongue.

(D) It receives general visceral afferent (GVA) inputs from the carotid sinus.

(E) Special visceral efferent (SVE) fibers of this nerve innervate the stylopharyngeus muscle.

306. Lesions of the vagus nerve may result in all of the following EXCEPT:

(A) hoarseness

(B) difficulty in swallowing

(C) a transient bradycardia

(D) loss of the baroreceptor reflex

(E) death when the lesion is bilateral

307. Interruption of the fibers of the glossopharyngeal nerve will produce all of the following signs or symptoms EXCEPT:

(A) loss of the gag reflex

(B) loss of taste sensation from the posterior third of the tongue

(C) difficulties in swallowing

(D) loss of the carotid sinus reflex

(E) dysphonia

308. All of the following statements concerning corticobulbar fibers are true EXCEPT:

(A) They are distributed to sensory relay nuclei.

(B) They arise principally from the precentral and postcentral gyri.

(C) They are distributed primarily (if not exclusively) to nuclei of the contralateral side.

(D) They are distributed to motor nuclei of cranial nerves.

(E) They extensively innervate several nuclei of the reticular formation.

309. Lesions involving the dorsolateral medulla can produce:

(A) loss of pain and thermal sensation on contralateral half of the face

(B) loss of pain and temperature sensation on ipsilateral side of the body

(C) dysphonia

(D) hemiparesis

(E) intention tremor

310. Nuclei or fibers present at the level of the cerebellopontine angle include all of the following cranial nerves EXCEPT:

(A) cochlear

(B) abducens

(C) facial

(D) glossopharyngeal

(E) vestibular

311. Which of the following statements concerning the olivocochlear bundle is correct:

(A) It arises from the inferior olivary nucleus and projects to the cochlea.

(B) Stimulation of it inhibits acoustic fiber responses to auditory stimuli.

(C) It communicates directly with the medial lemniscus.

(D) It can be seen easily in brainstem sections taken from upper pons.

(E) It is part of the ascending auditory pathway to the dorsal cochlea nucleus

312. Components of the auditory system include all of the following EXCEPT:

(A) spiral ganglia

(B) dorsal cochlear nucleus

(C) trapezoid body

(D) inferior olivary nucleus

(E) superior olivary nucleus

313. Unilateral deafness may result from a lesion of:

(A) the auditory cortex of one side

(B) the lateral lemniscus of one side

(C) cranial nerve VIII on one side

(D) medial geniculate

(E) medial lemniscus

314. Vestibular nuclei project to all of the following structures EXCEPT:

(A) spinal cord

(B) motor nucleus of cranial nerve VI

(C) motor nucleus of cranial nerve V

(D) motor nucleus of cranial nerve III

(E) cerebellum

315. Components of the facial nerve include all of the following EXCEPT:

(A) general somatic afferent fibers

(B) general somatic efferent fibers

(C) special visceral efferent fibers

(D) general visceral efferent fibers

(E) special visceral afferent fibers

316. Which of the following contain first-order sensory neurons with their cell bodies located within the central nervous system:

(A) geniculate ganglion

(B) spiral ganglion

(C) mesencephalic nucleus of cranial nerve V

(D) solitary nucleus

(E) Scarpa's ganglia

317. A lesion of cranial nerve VII proximal to its entry into the central nervous system will produce all of the following deficits EXCEPT:

(A) impairment of lacrimation on the side of the lesion

(B) complete loss of taste over the anterior part of the tongue

(C) hyperacusis

(D) loss of the corneal reflex on the side of the lesion

(E) increased difficulty in swallowing

318. In a lateral gaze paralysis, both eyes are conjugatively directed to the side opposite the lesion. In this condition, the locus of the lesion is:

(A) root fibers of cranial nerve III

(B) nucleus of cranial nerve III

(C) root fibers of cranial nerve VI

(D) nucleus of cranial nerve VI

(E) nucleus and root fibers of cranial nerve IV

319. Concerning the paramedian pontine reticular formation:

(A) it projects fibers directly to the hypoglossal nucleus

(B) bilateral lesions cause a partial deafness

(C) it projects its fibers to the basal ganglia

(D) it is a critical site for the integration of impulses regulating vertical and horizontal gaze

(E) it is a major site of noradrenergic fibers that project to the forebrain

320. A patient displays an ipsilateral paralysis of lateral gaze coupled with a contralateral hemiplegia. A lesion is most likely situated in the:

(A) ventromedial medulla

(B) dorsomedial medulla

(C) ventrocaudal pons

(D) dorsorostral pons

(E) ventromedial midbrain

321. Which of the following cranial nerves all carry special visceral afferent fibers:

(A) V, VII, and IX

(B) III, VI, and XII

(C) IX, X, and XI

(D) II, VII, and VIII

(E) I, VII, and IX

322. A patient displays the following constellation of symptoms: upper motor neuron paralysis of the left leg, paralysis of the lower half of the left side of the face, and a left homonymous hemianopsia. The lesion is most likely located in the:

(A) medulla

(B) basilar pons

(C) pontine tegmentum

(D) midbrain

(E) forebrain

323. A patient is unable to move his eyes downward. The lesion is most likely situated in the:

(A) medulla

(B) basilar aspect of the pons

(C) pontine tegmentum

(D) midbrain

(E) cerebellum

324. A patient is capable of displaying pupillary constriction during an accommodation reaction but not in response to a direct light stimulus. The lesion is most likely present in the:

(A) optic nerve

(B) ventral cell column of cranial nerve III

(C) pretectal area

(D) visual cortex

(E) Edinger-Westphal nucleus of cranial nerve III

325. Structures associated with the taste pathway include:

(A) geniculate ganglion, chorda tympani, and medial lemniscus

(B) solitary nucleus, parabrachial nucleus, and ventral posteromedial nucleus

(C) solitary nucleus, ventral posterolateral nucleus, and postcentral gyrus

(D) solitary nucleus, ventral posteromedial nucleus, and superior parietal lobule

(E) geniculate ganglion and ventral posterolateral nucleus

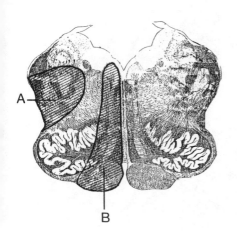

A—

B

(Adapted from Villiger, Fig. 10; with permission.)

Questions 326-331 Refer to the figure above.

326. The lesion at (A) would result from an occlusion of the:

(A) anterior spinal artery

(B) posterior inferior cerebellar artery

(C) superior cerebellar artery

(D) vertebral artery

(E) basilar artery

327. Structures affected by the lesion at (A) would include all of the following EXCEPT:

(A) spinothalamic fibers

(B) nucleus ambiguus

(C) nucleus solitarius

(D) lateral vestibular nucleus

(E) spinal tract of cranial nerve V

328. A lesion at (A) would produce all of the following dysfunctions EXCEPT:

(A) hoarseness

(B) loss of pharyngeal reflexes

(C) loss of pain and temperature sensation on the contralateral side of the face

(D) loss of pain and temperature sensation on the opposite side of the body

(E) Horner's syndrome

329. The lesion at (B) is most likely due to an occlusion of the:

(A) anterior spinal artery

(B) posterior inferior cerebellar artery

(C) superior cerebellar artery

(D) vertebral artery

(E) basilar artery

330. Structures affected by the lesion at (B) include all of the following EXCEPT:

(A) medial lemniscus

(B) medial longitudinal fasciculus

(C) nucleus solitarius

(D) hypoglossal nucleus

(E) pyramidal tract

331. A lesion at (B) would produce all of the following syndromes EXCEPT:

(A) contralateral hemiparesis

(B) contralateral loss of position sense

(C) ipsilateral hemiparalysis of tongue

(D) Horner's syndrome

(E) contralateral loss of vibration sense

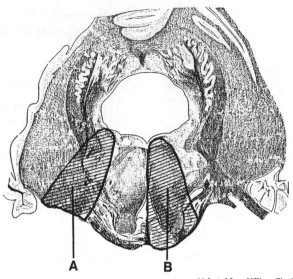

A   B

(Adapted from Villiger, Fig. 15; with permission.)

Questions 332-337 Refer to the figure above.

332. The lesion at (A) is most likely the result of an occlusion of the:

(A) vertebral artery

(B) anterior inferior cerebellar artery

(C) basilar artery

(D) anterior spinal artery

(E) posterior spinal artery

333. Structures affected by the lesion at (A) include all of the following EXCEPT:

(A) spinal nucleus of cranial nerve V

(B) fibers of cranial nerve VII

(C) spinothalamic fibers

(D) medial lemniscus

(E) vestibular nuclei

334. The lesion at (A) would most likely produce all of the following EXCEPT:

(A) ipsilateral facial paralysis

(B) ipsilateral limb ataxia

(C) loss of the gag reflex

(D) ipsilateral loss of cutaneous sensation of the face

(E) nerve deafness

335. The lesion at (B) is most likely the result of an occlusion of the:

(A) vertebral artery

(B) anterior inferior cerebellar artery

(C) basilar artery

(D) anterior spinal artery

(E) posterior spinal artery

336. Structures affected by the lesion at (B) include all of the following EXCEPT:

(A) medial lemniscus

(B) vestibular nuclei

(C) medial longitudinal fasciculus

(D) fibers of cranial nerve VII

(E) nucleus of cranial nerve VI

337. The lesion at (B) would produce all of the following deficits EXCEPT:

(A) paralysis of gaze to the side of the lesion

(B) paralysis of ipsilateral (lateral) rectus muscle

(C) contralateral hemiparesis

(D) ipsilateral loss of sensation to the face

(E) ipsilateral facial paralysis

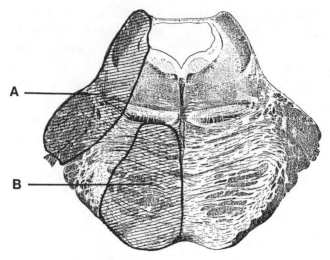

(Adapted from Villiger, Fig. 18; with permission.)

Questions 338-343 Refer to the figure above.

338. The lesion at (A) most likely resulted from an occlusion of the:

(A) basilar artery

(B) superior cerebellar artery

(C) anterior spinal artery

(D) vertebral artery

(E) posterior inferior cerebellar artery

339. Structures affected by the lesion at (A) include all of the following EXCEPT:

(A) spinothalamic fibers

(B) lateral lemniscus

(C) locus ceruleus

(D) motor nucleus of cranial nerve V

(E) spinal nucleus of cranial nerve V

340. The lesion at (A) results in all of the following deficits EXCEPT:

(A) nystagmus

(B) ipsilateral loss of masticatory reflexes

(C) diminution of hearing

(D) Horner's syndrome

(E) loss of pain and temperature sensation from the contralateral side of the body

341. The lesion at (B) is most likely the result of an occlusion of the:

(A) paramedian branch of the basilar artery

(B) circumferential branch of the basilar artery

(C) superior cerebellar artery

(D) anterior inferior cerebellar artery

(E) anterior spinal artery

342. Structures affected by the lesion at (B) include:

(A) medial lemniscus

(B) lateral lemniscus

(C) corticospinal tract

(D) medial longitudinal fasciculus

(E) tectospinal tract

343. The lesion at (B) would most likely result in which of the following deficits:

(A) paralysis of the contralateral limbs

(B) loss of conscious proprioception of the contralateral side of the body

(C) nystagmus

(D) lateral gaze paralysis

(E) facial paralysis

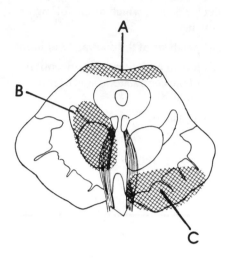

A

B

C

(Adapted from Kandel, Figure 46-14; with permission.)

Questions 344-348 Refer to the figure above.

344. A patient with the lesion at (A) in Figure 16 will generally show which of the following deficits:

(A) partial blindness

(B) loss of ability to gaze medially

(C) loss of ability to show tracking movements

(D) loss of accommodation reflex

(E) nystagmus

345. Structures damaged by the lesion at (B) in Figure 16 include all of the following EXCEPT:

(A) red nucleus

(B) medial lemniscus

(C) lateral lemniscus

(D) cranial nerve III

(E) central tegmental field

346. Which of the following deficits is likely to occur as a result of the lesion at (B) in Figure 16:

(A) contralateral loss of conscious proprioception

(B) transient tremor of the ipsilateral limb

(C) ipsilateral fourth nerve palsy

(D) hearing loss

(E) contralateral loss of taste sensation

347. As a result of the lesion at (C) in Figure 16, a patient will display all of the following deficits EXCEPT:

(A) supranuclear paresis of lower facial muscles

(B) contralateral loss of conscious proprioception of the limbs

(C) ipsilateral cranial nerve III paralysis

(D) contralateral hemiplegia

(E) supranuclear paresis of tongue muscles

348. The deficits associated with the lesion at (C) in Figure 16 are the result of damage to:

(A) substantia nigra and crus cerebri

(B) red nucleus and crus cerebri

(C) crus cerebri and cranial nerve III

(D) red nucleus and substantia nigra

(E) substantia nigra and cranial nerve III

349. The principal ascending auditory pathway of the brainstem is:

(A) medial lemniscus

(B) lateral lemniscus

(C) trapezoid body

(D) trigeminal lemniscus

(E) brachium of the superior colliculus

350. Which of the following statements best describes the regions of the ventral tegmental area and pars compacta of the substantia nigra:

(A) Both regions contain dopaminergic neurons but project to different populations of forebrain structures.

(B) Both regions provide converging dopaminergic inputs to the hypothalamus.

(C) Both regions provide converging dopaminergic inputs to the neostriatum.

(D) Both regions are innervated by GABAergic fibers and project to the cerebral cortex.

(E) Lesions of either region result in the development of a Parkinsonian-like syndrome.

The Brainstem
and Cranial Nerves

Answers

216-228. The answers are: 216-C, 217-E, 218-D, 219-E, 220-B, 221-A, 222-A, 223-E, 224-F, 225- E, 226- A, 337-A, 228-E. (Wilson-Pauwels, pp. VIII, 26, 50, 83, 98-101, 107-110, 114, 126) The mesencephalic nucleus of cranial nerve V receives inputs from the head associated with unconscious proprioception (general somatic afferent) (C). The otic ganglion contains postganglionic parasympathetic neurons (in association with cranial nerve IX) that innervate the parotid gland and is therefore classified as general visceral efferent (E). The nodose ganglion contains first-order cell bodies from cranial nerve IX and cranial nerve X which mediate inputs from visceral organs associated with chemoreceptors and baroreceptors and are thus classified as general visceral afferent (D) fibers. The pterygopalatine ganglion contains cells that constitute the postganglionic parasympathetic fibers for cranial nerve VII that innervate the lacrimal, nasal, and palatine glands. Accordingly, it is classified as general visceral efferent (E). The geniculate ganglion contains the first-order cell bodies associated with fibers of cranial nerve VII that mediate taste (special visceral afferent) (B) information to the solitary nucleus of the brainstem. The spiral ganglion and Scarpa's (vestibular) ganglion contain the cell bodies of first-order auditory and vestibular fibers, respectively, that pass to the lower brainstem. These neurons are classified as special somatic afferent (A). The superior salivatory nucleus contains preganglionic parasympathetic neurons for cranial nerve VII that make synaptic contact with neurons in the pterygopalatine and submandibular ganglia and are thus classified as general visceral efferent (E). The motor nucleus of cranial nerve V innervates the muscles of mastication and, since it is derived from the first branchial arch, it is classified as a special visceral efferent (F) nerve. The Edinger-Westphal nucleus of cranial nerve III projects its axons to the ciliary ganglion, whose fibers in turn innervate the ciliary muscles (activation induces the lens to bulge for accommodation) or to the pupillary constrictor muscles for pupillary constriction. Since these are both smooth muscles, the Edinger-Westphal cells constitute preganglionic parasympathetic neurons and the ciliary ganglion cells, postganglionic parasympathetic neurons. Each is classified as general visceral efferent (E). The superior vestibular nucleus receives direct inputs from first-order vestibular neurons and the optic nerve contains fibers whose origin is retinal ganglion cells. Accordingly, both of these structures are classified as special somatic afferent (A).

229-244.   The answers are: 229-E, 230-C, 231-H, 232-E, 233-A, 234-J, 235-K, 236-D, 237-B, 238-O, 239-N, 240-P, 241-I, 242-A, 243-G, 244-A. (Carpenter and Sutin, 8th Ed., pp. 316-357) The nucleus ambiguus (E) gives rise to lower motor neurons of cranial nerves IX and X. Fibers associated with cranial nerve IX innervate pharyngeal muscles. Preganglionic parasympathetic neurons of cranial nerve IX arise from the inferior salivatory nucleus (C) and make synapse in the optic ganglion. Surgical destruction of the descending tract of cranial nerve V (H) has been utilized to eliminate facial pain. The nucleus ambiguus (E) also gives rise to axons that comprise part of cranial nerve X that innervate laryngeal muscles. The solitary nucleus (A) receives first-order baroreceptor afferents from cranial nerves IX and X. The descending tract of the medial longitudinal fasciculus (MLF) arises from the medial vestibular nucleus (J), while stimulation of the lateral vestibular nucleus (K) facilitates extensor motor neurons. Baroreceptors are located in the carotid sinus (D), and the afferent processes have their cell bodies located in the inferior ganglion (O). The dorsal motor nucleus of the vagus (B) gives rise to preganglionic parasympathetic fibers that comprise the descending vagus and which cause slowing of heart rate upon stimulation. The external ear is innervated by general somatic afferent (GSA) fibers of cranial nerve IX that have their cell bodies in the superior ganglion (N). Axons of cells located in the otic ganglion (P) are postganglionic parasympathetics that innervate the parotid gland for controlling salivation. Climbing fibers arising from the inferior olivary nucleus (I) make synaptic contact with dendrites of Purkinje cells. Stimulation of the inferior olivary nucleus directly excites Purkinje cells, causing these neurons to discharge. The efferent pathways of the cerebellum arise from several nuclear groups. One such nucleus is the dentate nucleus (G). In addition to participating in cardiovascular functions, the solitary nucleus (A) is a major relay nucleus for the taste system. One of the primary target structures of this nucleus with respect to the taste pathway is the ventral posteromedial nucleus (VPM) of the thalamus.

245-249.   The answers are: 245-E, 246-B, 247-C, 248-D, 249-A. (Carpenter and Sutin, 8th Ed., pp. 381-385, 431) A lesion situated in the right dorsomedial pons, caudally (E), will affect the nucleus of cranial nerve VI along with surrounding tissue. This will invariably include the fibers of cranial nerve VII which wrap around the nucleus of cranial nerve VI. As a result, there will be a loss of both facial expression on the right side, because cranial nerve VII innervates the muscles of facial expression, along with an inability to move the right eye laterally, because cranial nerve VI innervates the lateral rectus muscle. Cranial nerve III innervates all of the rectus muscles except the lateral rectus. Therefore, a patient sustaining a lesion of this nerve will not be able to move the eye on the affected side medially (B). The fourth cranial nerve (C) innervates the superior oblique muscle which moves the eye downward from a medial position. This most often occurs when walking down a flight of stairs. A lesion of the right medial longitudinal fasciculus (D) will disrupt axons arising from the nucleus of cranial nerve VI of the left side that cross over and ascend to the occulomotor complex. Thus, this lesion would produce a dissociation of horizontal eye movements in which gazing to the left would result in a paresis of right ocular adduction together with monocular horizontal nystagmus in the left (abducting) eye.

250-254. The answers are: 250-A, 251-B, 252-E, 253-C, 254-D. (Carpenter and Sutin, 8th Ed., pp. 316-325) The nucleus gracilis (A) contains cells that respond to movement of the lower limb as a result of joint capsule activation. The nucleus cuneatus (B) contains cells that respond to a variety of stimuli applied to the upper limb, including vibratory stimuli. One component of the descending medial longitudinal fasciculus (MLF) (E) contains fibers that arise from the medial vestibular nucleus that projects to cervical levels and which contribute to reflex activity associated with the position of the head. Fibers of the medial lemniscus (D) arise from the contralateral dorsal column nuclei and ascend to the ventral postero-lateral nucleus (VPL) of the thalamus. These fibers transmit the same information noted above for the dorsal column nuclei which include, in part, 2-point discrimination and conscious proprioception from the opposite side of the body.

255-263. The answers are: 255-B, 256-C, 257-H, 258-B, 259-H, 260-G, 261-I, 262-A, 263-E. (Carpenter and Sutin, 8th Ed., pp. 330-352) Fibers contained in the inferior cerebellar peduncle (E) arise from cells located in both the spinal cord and brainstem. Different groups of neurons in the solitary complex (B) respond to taste stimuli and to inputs signaling sudden changes in blood pressure. The medial vestibular nucleus (C) receives direct vestibular inputs from the otolith organ and semicircular canals. Axons of medial vestibular neurons descend to the spinal cord in the medial longitudinal fasciculus (MLF) and serve to regulate reflexes associated with the head. The inferior olivary nucleus (H) receives inputs from the red nucleus and spinal cord, and it projects its axons to the contralateral cerebellar cortex where they synapse with the dendrites of Purkinje cells. The nucleus ambiguus (G) is the only special visceral efferent (SVE) structure labeled in this diagram and is situated lateral to the position occupied by the hypoglossal nucleus (A), which is the only general somatic efferent (GSE) structure labeled. Damage to the pyramids (I) results in an upper motor neuron paralysis since fibers of the corticospinal tract are disrupted.

264-269. The answers are: 264-A, 265-B, 266-A, 267-C, 268-A, 269-C. (Carpenter and Sutin, 8th Ed., pp. 470-474) The dentate nucleus (C) projects fibers to the ventrolateral (VL) nucleus of the thalamus and constitutes an important link in a feedback pathway to the cerebral cortex (VL projects to layer 4 of the cortex). The dentate nucleus also receives inputs from Purkinje cells located in the lateral aspect of the cerebellar cortex. The fastigial nucleus (A) receives its inputs from Purkinje cells of the medial (vermal) aspect of the cerebellar cortex and projects to the reticular formation and vestibular nuclei. Regulation of motor functions associated with the axial musculature is functionally associated with the vermal region of cerebellar cortex and the fastigial nucleus. Since the fastigial nucleus also provides a significant input into the vestibular nuclei, which, in turn, provides critical inputs to the ascending component of the medial longitudinal fasciculus (MLF) for regulation of eye movements, damage to the fastigial region will likely disrupt the inputs into the MLF and result in nystagmus. Neurons of the emboliform (B) and adjoining globose (not labeled) nucleus, sometimes referred to as interposed nuclei because of their intermediate position between the fastigial and dentate nuclei, project their axons to the red nucleus.

270-276. The answers are: 270-B, 271-E, 272-D, 273-A, 274-G, 275-F, 276-C. (Carpenter and Sutin, 8th Ed., p. 349, Fig. 11-28, pp. 330-357) The inferior vestibular nucleus (B) lies immediately medial to the inferior cerebellar peduncle (C) and receives direct inputs from first-order vestibular fibers. The medial longitudinal fasciculus (E) contains second-order vestibular fibers that mostly ascend to cranial nerves III, IV, and VI but which also descend to spinal levels. The solitary nucleus (D) receives inputs from first-order neurons mediating both taste (special visceral afferent) and cardiovascular (general visceral afferent) information. The hypoglossal nucleus (A) projects its axons to both extrinsic and intrinsic muscles of the tongue. The medial lemniscus (G) ascends to the thalamus and transmits information associated with conscious proprioception. The spinal nucleus of cranial nerve V (F) receives pain and temperature fibers from first-order trigeminal neurons from the head. The inferior cerebellar peduncle (C) is one of two principal cerebellar afferent pathways. One major fiber group contained within the inferior cerebellar peduncle arises from the contralateral inferior olivary nucleus.

277-281. The answers are: 277-C, 278-B, 279-D, 280-A, 281-E. (Carpenter and Sutin, 8th Ed., pp. 391-402) The middle cerebellar peduncle (C) serves as a relay nucleus for the transmission of information from the cerebral cortex to the cerebellum. Fibers in this peduncle arise from the contralateral deep pontine nuclei which receives its principal afferents from the cerebral cortex. The motor nucleus of cranial nerve V (B) is a lower motor neuron (special visceral efferent) because it innervates the muscles of mastication. Corticobulbar and corticospinal fibers (D) are situated in the ventral aspect of the basilar pons. Fibers of the superior cerebellar peduncle (A) project to both the red nucleus and ventrolateral nucleus (VL) of the thalamus. The medial lemniscus (E) is a somatotopically organized pathway that arises from the dorsal column nuclei and projects to the ventral posterolateral (VPL) nucleus of the thalamus. Fibers of this pathway that arise from the nucleus gracilis (associated with the leg) project to more dorsolateral aspects of the VPL. Fibers arising from the nucleus cuneatus (associated with the arm) project to more ventromedial aspects of the VPL.

282-286. The answers are: 282-E, 283-B, 284-C, 285-A, 286-D. (Carpenter and Sutin, 8th Ed., pp. 410-417) The inferior colliculus (E) is situated in the caudal aspect of the tectum and is an important relay nucleus for the transmission of auditory information to the cortex from lower levels of the brainstem. The decussation of the superior cerebellar peduncle (B) is also present at caudal levels of the midbrain and is usually seen together with the inferior colliculus. These crossing fibers arise from the dentate and interposed nuclei and terminate in the contralateral red nucleus and ventrolateral nucleus (VL) of the thalamus. The crus cerebri (C) contains fibers arising from all regions of the cortex and projecting to all the levels of the brainstem and the spinal cord. The trochlear nucleus (cranial nerve IV) (A), which is situated just below the periaqueductal gray (E) at the level of the inferior colliculus, receives direct inputs from ascending fibers of the medial longitudinal fasciculus which arise from vestibular nuclei. The midbrain periaqueductal gray (D) contains dense quantities of enkephalin-positive cells and nerve terminals. This transmitter (or neuromodulator) plays an important role in the regulation of pain and emotional behavior.

287-291. The answers are: 287-E, 288-D, 289-A, 290-C, 291-F. (Carpenter and Sutin, 8th Ed., pp. 417-439) The superior colliculus (E), situated at a more rostral level of the tectum, plays an important role in tracking or pursuit of moving stimuli. The medial geniculate nucleus (D), which is part of the forebrain, actually sits over the lateral aspect of the midbrain and can be seen at rostral levels of the midbrain. It is part of an auditory relay system and receives its inputs from the inferior colliculus via fibers of the brachium of the inferior colliculus. The pars compacta is situated in the medial aspect of the substantia nigra (A) and contains dopamine neurons whose axons innervate the striatum. The red nucleus (C), a structure associated with motor functions, receives direct inputs from both the cerebral cortex and the cerebellum. The occulomotor nerve (cranial nerve III) (F), located at the level of the superior colliculus, contains general somatic efferent (GSE) components that innervate extraocular eye muscles and general visceral efferent (GVE) components whose postganglionic fibers innervate smooth muscles associated with pupillary constriction and bulging of the lens.

292. The answer is B. (Carpenter and Sutin, 8th Ed., pp. 282-289, 316-320) The fibers passing through the pyramidal decussation arise from areas 4,6, 3,1, and 2 (i.e., primary motor, premotor, and primary sensory regions) of the cerebral cortex. This bundle, situated at the most caudal aspect of the medulla, characterizes that level of the medulla. The descending fibers pass to all levels of the cord and provide the anatomical substrate underlying voluntary control of movements of the limbs. Thus, if the entire bundle of fibers contained within the decussation were destroyed, bilateral cortical inputs to spinal cord motor neurons governing both the arms and legs would be eliminated, and quadriplegia would result.

293. The answer is C. (Carpenter and Sutin, 8th Ed., pp. 265-270; Kandel, 3rd Ed., pp. 360-362, 378-380) The dorsal column nuclei contain first-order neurons that receive their principal inputs from the periphery of the ipsilateral side of the body and which ascend directly through the dorsal columns without interruption. Dorsal column nuclei are somatotopically organized. Their axons form the medial lemniscus which ascends contralaterally to the ventral posterolateral nucleus of the thalamus. Dorsal column neurons typically respond to one modality of sensation (e.g., either discriminating tactile or kinesthetic sensation) but not to both. In this manner, such neurons are functionally segregated at the level of the dorsal column nuclei. This property also continues at higher synaptic regions of this pathway including neurons situated in the ventral posterior lateral nucleus and the postcentral gyrus.

294. The answer is D. (Carpenter and Sutin, 8th Ed., pp. 265-273, 317-350) The fasciculus cuneatus and fasciculus gracilis are first-order sensory fibers that transmit information concerning conscious proprioception, vibration sensibility, tactile sensation, and 2-point discrimination from the upper and lower limbs ipsilaterally to the lower medulla. The spinal tract of cranial nerve V contains first-order somatosensory neurons that descend from their point of entrance into the brain to the lower medulla. Likewise, the fasciculus solitarius contains first-order fibers mediating, in part, taste impulses from all parts of the tongue and epiglottis. External arcuate fibers arise from a small nucleus called the arcuate nucleus located in the ventral aspect of the lower medulla; these fibers pass in a dorsolateral direction to enter the inferior cerebellar peduncle.

295. The answer is A. (Carpenter and Sutin, 8th Ed., pp. 323-325) The spinal trigeminal nucleus receives its sensory inputs from first-order neurons contained in the ipsilateral descending tract of cranial nerve V. A central property of the nucleus caudalis of the spinal trigeminal nucleus is that it is uniquely associated with pain inputs (to the exclusion of other parts of the trigeminal complex such as the main sensory nucleus and mesencephalic nucleus). Fibers from this nucleus mainly project contralaterally to the ventral posteromedial nucleus (VPM) of the thalamus.

296. The answer is C. (Carpenter and Sutin, 8th Ed., pp. 326-328; Kandel, 3rd Ed., pp. 1055-1056) The area postrema is of interest because it is a circumventricular organ associated with emetic functions. As a circumventricular organ, the area postrema constitutes a part of the ependymal lining of the brain's ventricular system (in this case, the fourth ventricle). The area postrema contains both fenestrated and nonfenestrated capillaries that allow for enhanced transport which possibly accounts for the fact that it lies outside the blood-brain barrier. Axons and dendrites from neighboring structures (but not from the forebrain) innervate this structure, which is composed of astroblast-like cells, arterioles, sinusoids, and some neurons. Various peptides (but not monoamine containing neurons) have also been shown to be present in this structure. Experimental evidence has strongly implicated the area postrema as a chemoreceptor trigger zone for emesis. It responds to digitalis glycosides and apomorphine.

297. The answer is D. (Carpenter and Sutin, 8th Ed., pp. 328-330) Recent histochemical and immunocytochemical data provide evidence that all of the transmitters listed, except dopamine, are present in different regions of the medulla. There is evidence that different cells situated in the lateral reticular nucleus of the ventrolateral medulla contain norepinephrine, epinephrine, or acetylcholine. These chemically identified neurons are also located in other regions of the medulla as well as in the reticular formation. Acetylcholine receptors and acetylcholinesterase-containing cells have been found in cranial nerve motor nuclei. Enkephalin-containing neurons have been identified in the region of the reticular formation adjacent to the nucleus raphe magnus, in the solitary nucleus, and in the spinal nucleus of cranial nerve V. Dopamine-containing cells are located in the midbrain but not in the medulla.

298. The answer is E. (Carpenter and Sutin, 8th Ed., pp. 332-335) The cerebral cortex and cerebellum contribute significant input to the medullary reticular formation. These play important roles in the regulation of motor functions. The reticular formation also receives inputs from a number of sensory systems. One source includes collaterals of spinothalamic fibers. A second source includes synaptic contacts with cranial nerve sensory nuclei such as the vestibular complex and spinal nucleus of nerve V. These inputs are of importance with respect to the activating properties of the reticular formation whereby excitability levels of cerebral cortical cells are enhanced. On the other hand, spinocerebellar fibers project uninterrupted directly to the anterior lobe of the cerebellum and do not have any collaterals that synapse in any part of the reticular formation. In fact, dorsal spinocerebellar fibers pass in the far dorsolateral aspect of the lower medulla and enter the inferior cerebellar peduncle where that structure is formed. This places the dorsal spinocerebellar tract in a position considerably removed from any part of the reticular formation.

299. The answer is E. (Carpenter and Sutin, 8th Ed., pp. 280, 330-332) One of the most important feature of the inferior olivary nucleus is that it serves as a relay nucleus connecting structures situated in various parts of the neuraxis with the cerebellum. These structures include the cerebral cortex, red nucleus of the midbrain, and ascending fibers from the spinal cord. Ascending fibers from the spinal cord are somatotopically organized and are activated by cutaneous afferents and group 1b afferents. Fibers passing to the cerebellum from the inferior olivary nucleus end as climbing fibers (upon the dendritic trees of Purkinje neurons) and not as mossy fibers.

300. The answer is C. (Carpenter and Sutin, 8th Ed., pp. 334-335) Cells situated in the lateral third of the reticular formation generally constitute the receiving area for inputs from different regions of the central nervous system. These cells typically give rise to short axons that project to neighboring regions of the reticular formation. The major descending and ascending fibers arise from nuclei situated in the medial third of the medullary reticular formation. Descending fibers project to the spinal cord for inhibition of spinal motor neurons and spinal reflexes, while ascending fibers project to a wide variety of forebrain structures. In addition, fibers arising from a part of the medial aspect of the medullary reticular formation (paramedian nucleus) project to the vermal region of the anterior lobe of the cerebellum. Fibers from the median raphe nuclei synthesize serotonin, and these fibers project to the spinal cord, in part, for the regulation of pain sensation.

301. The answer is C. (Wilson-Pauwels, Cranial Nerves (Sandoz Course), B.C. Decker, Inc., Toronto, 1988, p. VIII) Cranial nerves XII, III, IV, and VI contain motor components that are categorized as general somatic efferent fibers (GSE), which means that they innervate structures derived from myotomes. In contrast, the motor component of the trigeminal nerve innervates structures derived from the first branchial arch and is thus called a special visceral efferent (SVE) nerve. The term "visceral" has been retained because the branchial arches are gill arches in fish, and these muscles are associated with visceral functions such as eating and breathing (gas exchange).

302. The answer is B. (Wilson-Pauwels, pp. 148-149) Activation of the hypoglossal nerve causes the tongue to point to the opposite side. Thus, a lesion of the lower motor neuron (i.e., the hypoglossal nucleus, situated in the dorsomedial aspect of the medulla, or hypoglossal nerve) will cause the tongue to be deviated to the side of the lesion (due to the unopposed action of the muscles of the same side whose innervation is intact). Upper motor neurons from the cerebral cortex innervate the hypoglossal nucleus of the opposite side. Because these fibers are crossed, a lesion of the upper motor neuron will produce an effect opposite to that observed when the lower motor neuron is damaged. Such a lesion will result in fasciculation of the tongue but will not cause the tongue to atrophy because these muscles are still innervated by an intact hypoglossal nerve. In contrast, damage to the hypoglossal nerve will cause a lower motor neuron paralysis in which the affected muscles will display atrophy.

303. The answer is E. (Wilson-Pauwels, pp. 140-145) The cell bodies of the accessory nerve are situated in the lateral aspect of the upper 5 or 6 segments of the anterior horn of the spinal cord. The axons of this nerve pass laterally out of the spinal cord and emerge as a series of rootlets. The fibers ascend and exit through the jugular foramen to innervate the sternomastoid and trapezius muscles. Lesions of the accessory nerve result in a downward and lateral rotation of the scapula and dropping of the shoulder due to the weakness of the trapezius muscle. An upward tilting of the head and its rotation to the opposite side will result from a lesion due in part to damage to the fibers that innervate the sternomastoid. Normally, contraction of the sternomastoid muscle causes the mastoid process to be pulled toward the clavicle, which leads to rotation of the head and its upward tilting to the contralateral side. There is no general somatic afferent component to this nerve.

304. The answer is A. (Wilson-Pauwels, pp. 126-137) Cranial nerve X is a highly complex nerve. It contains a few general somatic afferents from the back of the ear that enter the brain as cranial nerve X but terminate in the trigeminal complex. Special visceral afferents include fibers from chemoreceptors for taste associated with the epiglottis and chemoreceptors in the aortic bodies that sense changes in O_2-CO_2 levels in the blood. General visceral afferent fibers arise from the trachea, pharynx, larynx, and esophagus and signal changes in blood pressure to the brainstem. Special visceral efferent fibers innervate the constrictor muscles of the pharynx and the intrinsic muscles of the larynx. General visceral efferent fibers constitute part of the cranial aspect of the parasympathetic nervous system. Thus, they are preganglionic parasympathetic fibers that innervate the heart, lung, esophagus, and stomach.

305. The answer is A. (Wilson-Pauwels, pp. 114-123; Carpenter and Sutin, 8th Ed., pp. 350-352) There is a clear similarity between cranial nerves IX and X in that both contain a general visceral efferent (GVE) component. The only difference is that the GVE component of cranial nerve IX is composed of preganglionic parasympathetic neurons that synapse with postganglionic neurons innervating the parotid gland rather than structures regulating the cardiovascular system. Somatosensory inputs from the back of the ear (general somatic afferent) enter as cranial nerve IX but terminate within the trigeminal system. Special visceral afferent (SVA) components transmit information through cranial nerve IX into the brainstem including both taste (from the posterior third of the tongue) and changes in O_2-CO_2 levels in the blood (from the carotid body). General visceral afferent (GVA) fibers from the carotid sinus signal changes in blood pressure to the brainstem. Special visceral efferent (SVE) fibers from the brainstem innervate the stylopharyngeus muscle to elevate the upper pharynx and the upper pharyngeal constrictor muscle involved in swallowing.

306. The answer is C. (Wilson-Pauwels,, pp. 126-137, Carpenter and Sutin, 8th Ed., pp. 342-350) Lesions of the special visceral efferent (SVE) component of the vagus nerve can produces hoarseness as a result of damage to the recurrent laryngeal nerve which innervates the vocal cords. In addition, swallowing is made more difficult because of a paralysis of the pharyngeal constrictor muscles. Bradycardia will not occur. Instead, damage to the general visceral efferent (GVE) component of the vagus will cause a transient tachycardia, because of the unopposed action of the sympathetic nervous system. Since special visceral efferent (SVE) and general visceral efferent (GVE) fibers of the vagus constitute the efferent components of several reflex pathways such as the cough and baroreceptor reflexes, respectively, damage to these fibers will reduce or eliminate such reflexes. If the lesion is bilateral, death will likely ensue because of asphyxia. This is due to adduction of the vocal cords which obstructs air flow to the lungs.

307. The answer is E. (Wilson-Pauwels, pp. 114-135; Carpenter and Sutin, 8th Ed., pp. 349-352) While a pure lesion of cranial nerve IX is likely to be rare, it would produce a number of symptoms. These include: the loss of the gag (pharyngeal) reflex which involves constriction of the pharyngeal musculature and retraction of the tongue following tonsillar stimulation and difficulty in swallowing (both mediated by special visceral efferent fibers); loss of sensation from the posterior third of the tongue (mediated by special visceral afferent fibers); and loss of the carotid sinus reflex (mediated by special visceral afferent fibers of cranial nerve IX). Dysphonia (hoarseness) is a result of damage to the special visceral efferent fibers associated with the vagus nerve and not the glossopharyngeal.

308. The answer is C. (Carpenter and Sutin, 8th Ed., pp. 252-255) Corticobulbar fibers arise mainly from the precentral and postcentral gyri of the cerebral cortex and descend to all levels of the brainstem. Many of these fibers are bilaterally distributed to both sensory and motor cranial nerve nuclei. Only the descending fibers to cranial nerve XII and parts of VII (associated with lower jaw muscles) are crossed. Other descending fibers are distributed to several nuclear groups within the reticular formation.

309. The answer is C. (Carpenter and Sutin, 8th Ed., pp. 356-357) A primary characteristic of a lesion of the dorsolateral medulla is loss of pain and temperature sensation on the contralateral side of the body and ipsilateral half of the face. Damage to the descending tract of the trigeminal nerve and to the spinal nucleus of cranial nerve V will produce loss of sensation on the ipsilateral side of the face. There also will be damage to the lateral spinothalamic tract, which has already crossed at the level of the spinal cord, and which conveys pain and temperature sensation from the contralateral side of the body. In addition, fibers arising from the nucleus ambiguus exit laterally from the medulla, and these fibers, which innervate the larynx and pharynx, would also be affected causing dysphonia. Hemiparesis would not result from this lesion since the pyramidal tract would remain intact. The cerebellum would also be spared and intention tremor associated with cerebellar damage would not occur.

310. The answer is D. (Carpenter and Sutin, 8th Ed., pp. 356-357) The cerebellopontine angle is formed by the junction of the medulla, pons, and cerebellum. Cranial nerve nuclei or fibers present at this level include cranial nerve VIII (cochlear and vestibular components) and the facial and abducens nuclei. The glossopharyngeal nerve and associated nuclei such as the nucleus ambiguus and inferior salivatory nucleus are situated at more caudal levels of the medulla.

311. The answer is B. (Carpenter and Sutin, 8th Ed., pp. 371-374) The olivocochlear bundle is a most interesting pathway because it arises from the region immediately dorsal to the superior olivary nucleus and projects contralaterally back to the hair cells of the cochlea. Stimulation of this bundle results in inhibition or reduction of auditory nerve fiber responses to auditory signals. There is no evidence that the olivocochlear bundle bears any anatomical or functional relationship to the medial lemniscus. Since the pathway arises from the superior olivary nucleus which is present at the level of the lower pons, it would not be visible in a section taken from the upper pons.

312. The answer is D. (Carpenter and Sutin, 8th Ed., pp. 362-369) The cell bodies of first-order auditory fibers lie in the spiral ganglia. The dorsal cochlear nucleus receives first-order auditory fibers from the auditory nerve. The trapezoid body contains commissural auditory fibers which ascend to other auditory nuclei on the side contralateral to their entry. The superior olivary nucleus receives second-order auditory fibers from the ventral cochlear nucleus. In contrast, the inferior olivary nucleus is not a part of the auditory system but plays a central role in the regulation of cerebellar functions.

313. The answer is C. (Carpenter and Sutin, 8th Ed., p. 374) Since the auditory relay system is a highly complex pathway in which auditory signals are bilaterally represented at all levels beyond the receptor level, lesions at these levels would not produce a solely unilateral deafness. That could only result when the lesion involves either the receptor or the first-order neurons of the nerve (i.e., cranial nerve VIII itself). The medial lemniscus is not related to the auditory system.

314. The answer is C. (Carpenter and Sutin, 8th Ed., pp. 374-385) The lateral and medial vestibular nuclei project to different levels of the spinal cord. They also contribute fibers that pass through the medial longitudinal fasciculus to motor nuclei of cranial nerves III, IV, and VI. Moreover, fibers of the inferior and medial vestibular nuclei project to the cerebellum, and all four vestibular nuclei receive direct (first-order) neurons from the vestibular component of cranial nerve VIII. There are no known projections from the vestibular nuclei to the motor nucleus of cranial nerve V.

315. The answer is B. (Carpenter and Sutin, 8th Ed., pp. 385-389) The facial nerve is complex. It contains a few general somatic afferent (GSA) cutaneous fibers from the back of the ear and external auditory meatus as well as from muscle spindles in the muscles of facial expression. Special visceral efferent fibers (SVE) innervate the muscles of facial expression. General visceral efferent (GVE) fibers comprise the preganglionic parasympathetics that synapse with postganglionic sympathetic fibers that innervate the submandibular and sublingual salivary glands as well as the lacrimal gland and mucous membrane of the nose and mouth. Special visceral afferent (SVA) fibers comprise a major component of the taste system from the anterior third of the tongue. Since cranial nerve VII is associated with the second branchial arch, it has no general somatic efferent (GSE) component.

316. The answer is C. (Carpenter and Sutin, 8th Ed., p. 399) In general, first-order sensory neurons form ganglia outside the central nervous system. There is one exception — the mesencephalic nucleus of cranial nerve V, which transmits unconscious proprioception (i.e., muscle spindle activity) from jaw muscles. These inputs serve as the first-order neurons for a disynaptic pathway to the cerebellum as well as for a monosynaptic pathway with the motor nucleus of cranial nerve V for the jaw-closing reflex.

317. The answer is E. (Carpenter and Sutin, 8th Ed., pp. 385-389) A lesion of cranial nerve VII will produce impairment of lacrimation on the side of the lesion due to damage of the preganglionic parasympathetic fibers which synapse with postganglionics that innervate the lacrimal glands. Loss of taste over the anterior tongue is due to damage of the special visceral afferent fibers that mediate taste inputs to the central nervous system. Hyperacusis (marked increase in sensitivity or acuity to sounds) results from damage of fibers that normally supply the stapedius muscle whose function is to dampen oscillations of the ossicles. Loss of the corneal reflex on the side of the lesion occurs because the motor fibers that govern this reflex (i.e., cause the eyelid to close) are damaged. Difficulties in swallowing are caused by lesions of cranial nerve IX rather than cranial nerve VII.

318. The answer is D. (Carpenter and Sutin, 8th Ed., pp. 390-391) Conjugate lateral gaze requires the simultaneous contractions of the lateral rectus muscle of one eye and the medial rectus of the other eye. Recent studies have indicated that there is a region that integrates and coordinates such movements and that the site is part of the nucleus of cranial nerve VI. It is likely that it accomplishes this phenomenon, in part, because ascending axons from the abducens nucleus pass through the medial longitudinal fasciculus to the contralateral nuclei of cranial nerve III. Thus, the abducens nucleus serves not only to innervate the lateral rectus muscle but also to integrate signals necessary for conjugate deviation of the eyes. The abducens nucleus appears to be the only cranial nerve structure where lesions of the root fibers and nucleus fail to display identical effects.

319. The answer is D. (Carpenter and Sutin, 8th Ed., pp. 390-391) The paramedian pontine reticular formation is an important integrating structure controlling the position of the eyes. It receives inputs from the cerebral cortex (presumably the region of the frontal eye fields). It receives fibers from the cerebellum, spinal cord, and vestibular complex. Its efferent fibers project to the cerebellum, vestibular complex, pretectal region, interstitial nucleus of Cajal, and nucleus of Darkschewitsch of the rostral midbrain. These all are nuclei concerned with the regulation of eye position and movements. It is not related to any other known motor or auditory functions, nor has it been shown to contain ascending noradrenergic neurons.

320. The answer is C. (Carpenter and Sutin, pp. 380-392, 426-430) In order for a lesion to produce both an ipsilateral gaze paralysis and contralateral hemiplegia, it must be situated in a location where fibers regulating both lateral gaze and movements of the contralateral limbs lie close to each other. The only such location is the ventrocaudal aspect of the pons where fibers of cranial nerve VI descend toward the ventral surface of the brainstem and where corticospinal fibers are descending toward the spinal cord. The other regions listed in the question do not meet this condition.

321. The answer is E. (Wilson-Pauwels, p. VIII) The group called special visceral afferent fibers is limited to those cranial nerves that convey impulses to the brain associated with olfaction (I) and taste (VII, IX, and X). Since olfaction and taste involve chemical senses, some authors also include cranial nerves IX and X in the group because they contain components involved in signaling changes in O_2 and CO_2 levels in the blood.

322. The answer is E. (Carpenter and Sutin, 8th Ed., pp. 340-430, 544) Because the deficit includes a homonymous hemianopsia, the lesion has to be located somewhere in the forebrain, such as in the region that includes the optic tract and internal capsule on the right side of the brain. The motor neurons of cranial nerve VII as well as spinal cord motor neurons receive cortical fibers that are crossed, which accounts for the fact that motor dysfunctions of the lower face and body involve lesions on the same side.

323. The answer is D. (Wilson-Pauwels, pp. 26-47) Inability to move the eyes to a downward position may result from a lesion of cranial nerve IV (when the eye is positioned medially) or cranial nerve III (when the eye is positioned laterally). In either case, the cell bodies of origin of these cranial nerves are located in the midbrain.

324. The answer is C. (Carpenter and Sutin, 8th Ed., pp. 431-433) This disorder is referred to as the Argyll-Robertson pupil which occurs with central nervous system syphilis (tertiary). Although the precise site of the lesion has never been fully established, it is believed that its location is in the pretectal area. The reasoning is as follows: in the pupillary light reflex, many optic fibers terminate in the pretectal area and superior colliculus region and are then relayed to the autonomic nuclei of cranial nerve III. Impulses from this component of cranial nerve III then synapse with postganglionic parasympathetics that innervate the pupillary constrictor muscles, thus producing pupillary constriction. In the case of the accommodation reflex, retinal impulses first reach the cortex and are then relayed through corticofugal fibers to the brainstem. Some of these fibers are then relayed directly or indirectly to both motor and autonomic components of cranial nerve III, thus activating the muscles required for the accommodation reaction to occur, which includes pupillary constriction.

325. The answer is B. (Carpenter and Sutin, 8th Ed., pp. 385-389; Kandel, 3rd Ed., pp. 524-525) The solitary nucleus receives first-order neurons from the taste system and thus serves as a critical relay nucleus for the taste pathway. Axons arising from the solitary nucleus project to the ventral posteromedial nucleus of the thalamus and may also synapse in the parabrachial nuclei of the upper pons. Structures such as the ventral posterolateral nucleus, medial lemniscus, and superior parietal lobule are not associated with the taste pathway.

326. The answer is B. (Carpenter and Sutin, 8th Ed., p. 729; Kandel, 3rd Ed., pp. 726-727) At central levels of the medulla, its lateral aspect is supplied by the posterior inferior cerebellar artery. The anterior spinal artery supplies the ventral and dorsomedial aspects of this level of the medulla. The superior cerebellar and basilar arteries supply the dorsolateral and medial pons, respectively. The vertebral artery supplies intermediolateral portions of the medulla (just lateral to the regions supplied by the anterior spinal artery).

327. The answer is D. (Carpenter and Sutin, 8th Ed., p. 729; Kandel, 3rd Ed., pp. 726-727) Structures situated in the lateral aspect of central levels of the medulla include the nucleus ambiguus, whose axons innervate the muscles of the larynx and pharynx, spinothalamic fibers, which mediate pain and temperature signals from the contralateral side of the body, nucleus solitarius, whose afferents from higher centers are associated with autonomic (mainly sympathetic) functions, and the spinal tract of cranial nerve V, which mediates pain and temperature signals from the ipsilateral side of the face. The lateral vestibular nucleus is located in the dorsolateral aspect of the caudal pons and would not be affected by such a lesion.

328. The answer is C. (Carpenter and Sutin, p. 729; Kandel, 3rd Ed., pp. 726-727) Destruction of the lateral aspect of central levels of the medulla will affect special visceral efferent (SVE) fibers that innervate the pharynx and larynx and thus result in loss of pharyngeal reflexes and hoarseness. It will also affect ascending pain and temperature fibers associated with the contralateral side of the body and first-order pain and temperature fibers and cells associated with the ipsilateral (but not contralateral) side of the face. Also affected by the lesion at (A) are descending fibers from the hypothalamus and rostral brainstem that project to lower brainstem nuclei which integrate these outputs and, in turn, control autonomic functions. Damage to these descending forebrain and rostral brainstem fibers will typically produce a Horner's syndrome.

329. The answer is A. (Carpenter and Sutin, 8th Ed., p. 729; Kandel, 3rd Ed., pp. 726-727) The ventral and dorsomedial medulla are supplied by the anterior spinal artery. The vertebral artery supplies the region just lateral to that supplied by the anterior spinal artery. The posterior inferior cerebellar artery supplies the lateral aspect of the medulla, and the superior cerebellar and basilar arteries supply different parts of the pons.

330. The answer is C. (Carpenter and Sutin, 8th Ed., p. 729; Kandel, 3rd Ed., pp. 726-727) Structures situated within the ventromedial and dorsomedial aspects of central levels of the medulla include the medial lemniscus, medial longitudinal fasciculus, hypoglossal nucleus, and pyramidal tract. The nucleus solitarius, which mediates autonomic and taste functions, is situated in a more lateral position than the lesion and would thus not be affected by occlusion of the anterior spinal artery.

331. The answer is D. (Carpenter and Sutin, 8th Ed., p. 729; Kandel, 3rd Ed., pp. 726-727) The lesion shown at (B) would result in hemiparesis of the contralateral limbs from damage to the pyramidal tract, which crosses to the opposite side at lower levels of the central nervous system (i.e., the medulla-spinal cord border). There also would be loss of position and vibration sensation of the contralateral side because of damage to the medial lemniscus. This fiber bundle crosses at lower levels of the medulla and thus conveys these modalities of sensation from the opposite side of the body to higher centers of the brain. In addition, there would be an ipsilateral paralysis (i.e., hemiparalysis) of the tongue because the root fibers of the hypoglossal nerve on one side would be damaged. A Horner's syndrome would not likely occur because the descending fibers from higher centers and cell bodies within the medulla that regulate sympathetic functions are situated in a more lateral position within this level of the brainstem.

332. The answer is B. (Carpenter and Sutin, 8th Ed., pp. 728-729; Kandel, 3rd Ed., pp. 726-727) The lateral aspect of the lower pons is supplied by the anterior inferior cerebellar artery. The basilar artery supplies medial aspects of the pons, and the other arteries supply different parts of the medulla.

333. The answer is D. (Carpenter and Sutin, 8th Ed., pp. 728-729; Kandel, 3rd Ed., pp. 726-727) Structures situated in the lateral aspect of this level of the pons within the sphere of the lesion include the spinal nucleus of cranial nerve V, special visceral efferent fibers of cranial nerve VII, spinothalamic fibers, and vestibular nuclei. The medial lemniscus at this level of the pons is located medial to the lesion.

334. The answer is C. (Carpenter and Sutin, 8th Ed., pp. 728-729; Kandel, 3rd Ed., pp. 726-727) The lesion at (A) would result in: (1) an ipsilateral facial paralysis (damage to the facial nerve), (2) ipsilateral limb ataxia (damage to vestibular nuclei and fibers producing a cerebellar-like syndrome), (3) loss of ipsilateral facial cutaneous sensation (disruption of trigeminal fibers and spinal nucleus), and (4) nerve deafness (disruption of primary and secondary auditory fibers). The gag reflex would not be affected because it involves the nucleus ambiguus which is located at a more caudal level of the medulla.

335. The answer is C. (Carpenter and Sutin, 8th Ed., pp. 728-729; Kandel, 3rd Ed., pp. 726-727) The medial aspect of the pons is supplied by the basilar artery. The lateral aspect of the pons is supplied, in part, by the anterior inferior cerebellar artery. The vertebral, anterior spinal and posterior spinal arteries supply other regions of the medulla.

336. The answer is B. (Carpenter and Sutin, 8th Ed., pp. 728-729; Kandel, 3rd Ed., pp. 726-727) Structures situated in the medial aspect of the pons include the medial lemniscus, medial longitudinal fasciculus, nucleus of cranial nerve VI, and fibers of cranial nerve VII as they wrap around the nucleus of cranial nerve VI. Vestibular nuclei are situated in the dorsolateral aspect of the pons and, thus, would not be affected by this lesion.

337. The answer is D. (Carpenter and Sutin, 8th Ed., pp. 728-729; Kandel, 3rd Ed., pp. 726-727) The lesion at (B) would result in damage to the abducens nucleus and adjoining tissue, including the pontine gaze center, thus producing a paralysis of gaze to the side of the lesion and paralysis of the ipsilateral (lateral) rectus muscle. Because of damage to fibers of cranial nerve VII that wrap around the nucleus of cranial nerve VI, ipsilateral facial paralysis would also occur. A contralateral hemiparesis would be present because of damage to the pyramidal tract. There is little chance that such a lesion would produce ipsilateral loss of sensation to the face because the tract and cell bodies of the trigeminal system lie lateral to the position of the lesion.

338. The answer is B. (Carpenter and Sutin, 8th Ed., pp. 728-729) The superior cerebellar artery supplies the dorsolateral aspect of the upper pons. The basilar artery supplies the medial aspect of the pons. The other arteries (vertebral, anterior spinal and posterior inferior cerebellar) supply different parts of the medulla.

339. The answer is E. (Carpenter and Sutin, 8th Ed., pp. 728-729; Kandel, 3rd Ed., pp. 726-728) The lateral aspect of the upper pons contains spinothalamic fibers, the lateral lemniscus, and the locus ceruleus (situated just dorsal to the motor nucleus of cranial nerve V which is also affected by the lesion). The spinal nucleus of V would not be affected because it does not extend to the rostral pons.

340. The answer is A. (Carpenter and Sutin, 8th Ed., pp. 728-729; Kandel, 3rd Ed., pp. 726-727) This lateral pontine lesion produces a syndrome that includes: (1) loss of pain and temperature sensation from the contralateral side of the body (damage to the lateral spinothalamic tract), (2) ipsilateral loss of masticatory reflexes (damage to the motor nucleus of cranial nerve V), (3) diminution of hearing (disruption of secondary auditory pathways), and (4) Horner's syndrome (disruption of descending fibers from the hypothalamus and midbrain that mediate autonomic functions). Nystagmus would not occur because the medial longitudinal fasciculus is spared by the lesion.

341. The answer is A. (Carpenter and Sutin, 8th Ed., pp. 728-729; Kandel, pp. 726-728) The paramedian branch of the basilar artery supplies the ventromedial pons (i.e., medial basilar pons). The circumferential branch supplies more lateral regions of the pons as does the superior cerebellar artery. The anterior spinal and anterior inferior cerebellar arteries supply different parts of the medulla.

342. The answer is C. (Carpenter and Sutin, 8th Ed., pp. 728-729; Kandel, 3rd Ed., pp. 726-728) The lesion is restricted to the basilar pons. Thus, the only structure affected by this lesion among the choices given is the corticospinal tract. The other structures listed are situated in the tegmentum of the pons.

343. The answer is A. (Carpenter and Sutin, 8th Ed., pp. 728-729; Kandel, 3rd Ed., pp. 726-728) Since the lesion is restricted to the medial aspect of the basilar part of the pons, the corticospinal tract would be affected, producing a paralysis of the contralateral limbs. Although other structures would also be affected and could produce additional deficits, such deficits are not listed in this question. The other dysfunctions listed would not occur because they are associated with structures situated in the pontine tegmentum which is not included in this lesion.

344. The answer is C. (Carpenter and Sutin, 8th Ed., pp. 417-437; Kandel, 3rd Ed., pp. 728-729) The lesion involves the superior colliculus. This structure receives inputs from the cerebral cortex and optic tract and its neurons respond to moving objects in the visual field. It is considered essential for the regulation of tracking movements. Lesions of the superior colliculus have not been shown to produce any of the other deficits listed in this question. Nystagmus is not likely to occur because the lesion does not involve the medial longitudinal fasciculus or the pontine gaze center.

345. The answer is C. (Carpenter and Sutin, 8th Ed., pp. 417-437; Kandel, 3rd Ed., pp. 728-729) The lesion is basically situated in the tegmentum. Thus, it would damage fibers of cranial nerve III that pass through the tegmentum en route to its exit from the brain. The red nucleus, medial lemniscus, and central tegmental field would also be damaged. The lateral lemniscus is located in the far lateral midbrain at this level and, thus, it would not be affected by this lesion.

346. The answer is A. (Kandel, 3rd Ed., pp. 728-729) The lesion will disrupt fibers of the medial lemniscus (lateral aspect of the lesion) and thus produce contralateral loss of conscious proprioception. It will also disrupt fibers passing from the cerebellum to the red nucleus and ventrolateral (VL) nucleus of the thalamus which could account for a tremor of the contralateral limb. Note that there would be no ipsilateral motor loss because functions associated with the red nucleus are expressed on the contralateral side. Occulomotor palsy would also be present because the lesion disrupts root fibers of cranial nerve III. However, the lesion is too rostral to affect cranial nerve IV. There is no hearing loss because the auditory fibers are situated too far laterally. Since the taste pathway is essentially ipsilateral, if any fibers are damaged by the lesion, deficits in taste sensation would be ipsilateral.

347. The answer is B. (Carpenter and Sutin, 8th Ed., p. 436; Kandel, 3rd Ed., p. 728) The lesion is situated in the ventromedial aspect of the midbrain at the level of the superior colliculus. It will produce a supranuclear paresis of the lower facial and tongue muscles because the upper motor neurons (i.e., corticobulbar fibers) that innervate the motor neurons of cranial nerves VII and XII will be damaged. Damage to the corticospinal tract will result in contralateral hemiplegia. Since the occulomotor nerve exits medially, the lesion will also disrupt these fibers and cause an ipsilateral cranial nerve III paralysis. The lesion will not affect the medial lemniscus, since this structure is situated in a lateral position at this level of the brainstem.

348. The answer is C. (Carpenter and Sutin, 8th Ed., p. 436; Kandel, 3rd Ed., p. 728) The primary structures damaged by this lesion include the crus cerebri, which results in an upper motor neuron paralysis of the contralateral limbs as well as a paresis of the lower facial and tongue muscles. The other outstanding syndrome present from this lesion is a paralysis, resulting from damage to the cranial nerve III. While other structures may be marginally affected, they do not contribute to the syndrome present from such a lesion.

349. The answer is B. (Carpenter and Sutin, 8th Ed., pp. 372-373) The principal ascending pathway of the auditory system listed in this question is the lateral lemniscus. It transmits information from the cochlear nuclei to the inferior colliculus. The trapezoid body is a commissure which contains some of the fibers of the lateral lemniscus that cross from the cochlear nuclei of one side of the brainstem en route to the inferior colliculus of the other side. The trapezoid body is present at the level of the caudal pons. The brachium of the superior colliculus, trigeminal lemniscus, and medial lemniscus do not transmit auditory sensory information.

350. The answer is A. (Carpenter and Sutin, 8th Ed., pp. 444-451) The pars compacta of the substantia nigra contains dopamine neurons whose axons project to the neostriatum. In contrast, the dopaminergic neurons of the ventral tegmental area project to other areas of the forebrain, such as hypothalamus, limbic system, and cerebral cortex. There is no known overlap in the distribution of these dopaminergic projection systems. A Parkinsonian-like syndrome results from damage to the pars compacta of the substantia nigra, but not from a lesion restricted to the ventral tegmental region.

Sensory Systems

DIRECTIONS: The questions below consist of lettered headings followed by a set of numbered items. For each numbered item select the **one** heading with which it is **most** closely associated. Each lettered heading may be used **once, more than once, or not at all.**

Questions 351-356

    (A) horizontal cells
    (B) bipolar cells
    (C) ganglion cells
    (D) rods
    (E) cones
    (F) optic nerve fibers
    (G) Muller fibers
    (H) astrocytes

351. these processes arise from ganglion cells

352. an interneuron that allows for communication between a receptor cell and ganglion cell

353. concentrated in the fovea

354. a detector of dim light

355. these cells are capable of producing action potentials

356. capable of depolarizing photoreceptor cells

Questions 357-363

(A) emmetropia

(B) hyperopia

(C) myopia

(D) presbyopia

(E) astigmatism

(F) cataract

(G) glaucoma

357. light rays are focused in front of the retina

358. corrected with a cylindrical lens

359. corrected with a concave spherical lens

360. corrected with a convex lens

361. usually caused by an oblong shape of the cornea or lens

362. intraocular pressure is elevated due to a blockade of the canal of Schlemm

363. proteins of lens fibers become denatured and then coagulate

Questions 364-369

(A) left homonymous hemianopsia

(B) right homonymous hemianopsia

(C) bitemporal hemianopsia

(D) blindness in the right eye

(E) blindness in the left eye

(F) upper left quadrantanopia

(G) lower left quadrantanopia

(H) upper right quadrantanopia

(I) lower right quadrantanopia

364. lesion of the right optic nerve

365. lesion of the right temporal lobe

366. lesion of the right superior bank of the calcarine fissure

367. lesion of the right optic tract

368. lesion of the optic chiasm

369. lesion of the right inferior bank of the calcarine fissure

DIRECTIONS: Each question below contains five suggested responses. Select the **one best** response to each question

370. All of the following statements about the coding and processing of sensory information are correct EXCEPT:

(A) the sequence of connections associated with a given sensory process follows a hierarchical organization

(B) there usually exists a parallel processing system for the transmission of sensory information to the cortex

(C) sensory systems are somatotopically organized but not generally beyond the first synapse

(D) stimulus intensity may be encoded by the frequency of response by a given neuron

(E) stimulus intensity may be encoded by the numbers of neurons discharging

371. The conscious perception of movement is mediated by which of the following receptors:

(A) Meissner's corpuscles

(B) free nerve endings

(C) Merkel's receptors

(D) joint capsules

(E) pacinian corpuscles

372. One difference between rapidly adapting and slowly adapting receptors is:

(A) a rapidly adapting receptor responds continuously to the presence of a stimulus while a slowly adapting receptor responds only at the onset of the stimulus

(B) a rapidly adapting receptor responds only at the onset of the stimulus and to any step change in the stimulus position, while the slowly adapting receptor displays a persistent response to the presence of the stimulus

(C) a rapidly adapting receptor will not respond to any subsequent stimulus following the initial stimulus, while the slowly adapting receptor responds quite readily to a second stimulus

(D) a rapidly adapting receptor will discharge at a high frequency to the initial stimulus and then continue to discharge but at a somewhat lower rate, while a slowly adapting receptor will discharge at a high frequency throughout the period of the duration of the stimulus

(E) rapidly adapting receptors are limited to muscle spindles, while slowly adapting receptors include those associated with pain and temperature pathways

373. Meissner's corpuscles differ from pacinian corpuscles in all of the following ways EXCEPT:

(A) Meissner's corpuscles have small receptive fields while pacinian corpuscles have larger receptive fields

(B) Meissner's corpuscles can resolve fine spatial differences while pacinian corpuscles can only resolve coarse spatial differences

(C) Meissner's corpuscles are more sensitive to low frequency mechanical stimuli while pacinian corpuscles are more sensitive to high frequency stimuli

(D) Meissner's corpuscles have a less well developed perineural capsule than do pacinian corpuscles

(E) Meissner's corpuscles are slowly adapting receptors while pacinian corpuscles are rapidly adapting receptors

374. Which of the following types of inhibition have been identified within the dorsal column nuclei :

(A) feed forward inhibition utilizing local interneurons only

(B) feedback inhibition utilizing local interneurons only

(C) distal inhibition from fibers arising in the cerebral cortex only

(D) feed forward, feedback, and distal inhibition

(E) feed forward and distal inhibition only

375. All of the following statements concerning sensory receptors and neurons utilizing the dorsal column-medial lemniscal system are correct EXCEPT:

(A) The rate of adaptation will affect the way in which the stimulus will be perceived.

(B) Pacinian corpuscles represent an example of slowly adapting receptors.

(C) The discharge rate within a given neuron is a function of the intensity of the applied stimulus.

(D) A pressure receptor that maintains its response as long as the stimulus is applied is called a tonic receptor.

(E) Parallel pathways convey information to the cerebral cortex about different properties of a given stimulus.

376. As two stimuli are brought closer together spatially, one can still detect differences in the stimuli. This phenomenon is due to all of the following EXCEPT:

(A) two distinct zones of central excitation at each level of the sensory relay system

(B) high concentrations of receptors for that stimulus in the region of the body surface examined

(C) lateral inhibition

(D) the presence of an inhibitory feedback system that reaches to the receptor

(E) the presence of a somatotopically organized pathway

377. Neurons capable of responding to the direction or orientation of a given stimulus moved along a receptive field are located in:

(A) spinal cord

(B) medulla

(C) pons

(D) thalamus

(E) cerebral cortex

378. All the following play a role in the mediation or modulation of pain EXCEPT:

(A) neurons within the lateral hypo-thalamus

(B) substance P at primary afferent terminals

(C) opiate receptors in the spinal cord and brainstem

(D) neurons within the substantia gelatinosa

(E) neurons within the midbrain periaqueductal gray

379. Chemical mediators that can sensitize or activate the peripheral endings of nociceptors include all of the following EXCEPT:

(A) potassium

(B) enkephalins

(C) bradykinin

(D) histamine

(E) prostaglandins

380. Referred pain is the result of:

(A) Inhibitory fibers that block transmission of pain impulses along a given pathway which then get transferred to a different pathway associated with a different part of the body

(B) a massive discharge along a given pathway that results in the activation of a separate pathway because of the principle of divergence

(C) a convergence of primary afferent fibers from a given region onto second-order neurons that nor-mally receive primary afferents from a different body part

(D) the disruption of lateral spinotha-lamic fibers

(E) the blockade of substance P from primary afferent terminals

381. The terminals of different classes of primary nociceptive afferents have been shown to release which of the following transmitters onto dorsal horn neurons of the spinal cord:

(A) enkephalins alone

(B) glutamate alone

(C) substance P alone

(D) glutamate and substance P

(E) enkephalins, substance P, and glutamate

382. Structures known to receive nociceptive afferent fibers include all of the following EXCEPT:

(A) ventral posterolateral nucleus (VPL) of the thalamus

(B) lateral cervical nucleus of the spinal cord

(C) reticular formation of the medulla

(D) midbrain periaqueductal gray

(E) main sensory nucleus of cranial nerve V

383. Stimulation of gray matter around the cerebral aqueduct and fourth ventricle can produce analgesia. This phenomenon is explained in terms of:

(A) activation of a pathway that ascends directly to the cortex and which mediates analgesia

(B) a descending pathway that blocks nociceptive inputs at the level of the dorsal horn

(C) activation of local interneurons that block ascending nociceptive signals at the level of the midbrain

(D) activation of an ascending inhibitory pathway that projects to the ventral posterolateral nucleus (VPL) of thalamus

(E) activation of cholinergic neurons in the basal forebrain

384. The descending pathway for central control of nociception includes:

(A) fibers from the periaqueductal gray that synapse directly on dorsal horn cells

(B) fibers from the periaqueductal gray that synapse on neurons of the nucleus raphe magnus and these neurons then synapse on dorsal horn cells

(C) fibers from the periaqueductal gray that synapse upon inferior olivary neurons which then synapse upon dorsal horn cells

(D) hypothalamic fibers that synapse upon neurons of the nucleus solitarius which then synapse upon neurons of the dorsal horn

(E) hypothalamic fibers that synapse directly upon dorsal horn neurons

385. All of the following are true concerning the lateral geniculate nucleus EXCEPT:

(A) contains cells with circular, symmetrical receptive fields

(B) contains mostly relay cells that project to layer 4 of area 19 of the cerebral cortex

(C) receives afferents from the cerebral cortex

(D) receives contralateral retinal afferents which terminate on cells different from those which receive ipsilateral afferents from the retina

(E) receives a visuotopic projection from the retina

386. At the level of the dorsal horn of the spinal cord, nociceptive transmission may be blocked when descending fibers are:

(A) opioidergic and only contact dendrites of postsynaptic neurons that contain opiate receptors

(B) opioidergic and only contact opiate receptors located presynaptically on nociceptive terminals

(C) opioidergic and contact both dendrites of postsynaptic neurons and presynaptic terminals, both of which contain opiate receptors

(D) serotonergic and only contact dendrites of postsynaptic neurons that contain 5-HT receptors

(E) cholinergic and contact both dendrites of postsynaptic neurons and presynaptic terminals, both of which contain muscarinic receptors

387. All of the following statements concerning photoreceptors are correct EXCEPT:

(A) Outer segments of rods and cones contain densely packed visual pigments that are effective in absorbing light.

(B) Rods are specialized for day vision.

(C) Rods contain more photopigment and capture more light than cones.

(D) Discs of the outer segment are constantly being renewed.

(E) Absorption of light by visual pigments of photoreceptors leads to a change of ionic fluxes across the plasma membrane of the photoreceptor cells.

388. All of the following statements about events in the retina are correct EXCEPT:

(A) In the presence of light, 11-cis-Retinal is changed to all-trans-Retinal.

(B) In the presence of light, the rod cell becomes hyperpolarized.

(C) In the presence of light, there is a reduction of cyclicguanosine monophosphate (cyclic GMP) in the cytoplasm of the photoreceptor cell.

(D) In the presence of light, there is a closure of sodium channels.

(E) The flow of sodium into the photoreceptor cell is through cyclic GMP gated channels.

389. A cell that responds with an "on-center" and "off-surround" to generate contrast within the receptive field can be identified in:

(A) retina (ganglion cell)

(B) lateral geniculate nucleus

(C) retina (ganglion cell) and lateral geniculate nucleus

(D) layer 4 of the primary visual cortex (area 17)

(E) retina (ganglion cell), lateral geniculate nucleus, and area 18

390. When a cone is hyperpolarized by light:

(A) the "on-center" bipolar cell is excited and the "off-center" bipolar cell is inhibited

(B) the "on-center" bipolar cell will inhibit the ganglion cell with which it makes synaptic contact

(C) the ganglion cell which receives its input from an "off-center" bipolar cell will discharge because the bipolar cell is excited during the presence of the stimulus

(D) an "on-center" bipolar cell excites a neighboring ganglion cell which receives its input from an "off-center" bipolar cell

(E) transmitter released from a cone cell has the same effect upon all processes with which it synapses

391. Fibers in each optic tract synapse in:

(A) the lateral geniculate nucleus only

(B) the lateral geniculate nucleus and the pretectal area

(C) the lateral geniculate nucleus, the pretectal area, and the superior colliculus

(D) the lateral geniculate nucleus, the pretectal area, the superior colliculus, and the suprachiasmatic nucleus

(E) the lateral geniculate nucleus, the pretectal area, the superior colliculus, the suprachiasmatic nucleus, and the nuclei of cranial nerves III and IV

392. Lateral inhibition within the retina is most effectively achieved through the action of:

(A) rod cells

(B) cone cells

(C) bipolar cells

(D) ganglion cells

(E) horizontal cells

393. Anatomical relationships of the dorsolateral geniculate nucleus include all of the following EXCEPT:

(A) half of the fibers of each optic tract project to this nucleus on a given side, representing corresponding points on the two retinas

(B) fibers from the nasal retina project to the lateral geniculate of the same side and fibers from the temporal retina project to the lateral geniculate of the contralateral side

(C) layers II, III, and V receive inputs from the temporal retina while layers I, IV, and VI receive inputs from the nasal retina

(D) signals entering the lateral geniculate nucleus may be "gated" by descending fibers of the ipsilateral primary visual cortex

(E) layers I and II differ from the others in that they contain large cells which receive their inputs from Y retinal ganglion cells and serve as a rapidly conducting relay system to the cortex

394. Characteristics of layers III through VI of the lateral geniculate nucleus include all of the following EXCEPT:

(A) receive inputs from X cells of the retina

(B) communicate information concerning very accurate details of the visual field

(C) communicate visual information concerning color vision

(D) contain small- to medium-sized cells as compared with layers I and II

(E) receive collateral inputs from the hypothalamus

395. All of the following statements concerning the organization of the visual cortex are true EXCEPT:

(A) In the primary visual cortex, a given column may contain cells which display the same axis of orientation.

(B) The visual cortex contains sets of columns in which different cells respond to different orientations of a stimulus received by both eyes.

(C) The deepest part of layer 4 (i.e., layer 4c) may contain cells with concentric receptive fields whose axons project directly onto lateral geniculate cells as a feedback mechanism.

(D) A column may be specifically dedicated to the left or right eye.

(E) Cells within an ocular dominance column may lie in a specialized region (blob zone) that specifically responds to color signals.

396. All of the following statements concerning neural mechanisms related to color vision are true EXCEPT:

(A) Three different kinds of photo-chemicals are present in different cones causing a given cone to be selectively sensitive to one color.

(B) Retinal ganglion cells which receive their inputs from cone cells are unique in they do not display the concentric center-surround receptive field organization that is characteristic of ganglion cells that receive their inputs from rod cells.

(C) When information about color is transmitted by color opponent cells, it implies that a cell with a strong response to a light stimulus of green wavelength would be inhibited when a red light stimulus is presented.

(D) Single opponent cells are commonly found in both the retina and the lateral geniculate nucleus.

(E) Double opponent cells are found in blob zones of the visual cortex.

397. Cells that respond to an image in a specific position, have discrete excitatory and inhibitory zones, and a specific axis of orientation in which a response occurs are classified as:

(A) M cells of the lateral geniculate nucleus

(B) P cells of the lateral geniculate nucleus

(C) simple cells of the visual cortex

(D) complex cells of the visual cortex

(E) hypercomplex cells of the visual cortex

398. All of the following statements concerning the cochlea are true EXCEPT:

(A) High frequency sounds cause the basilar membrane to vibrate maximally at its base.

(B) Stereocilia from hair cells of the cochlea are attached to and embedded in the tectorial membrane.

(C) An endocochlear potential of +80 mV exists between the endolymph and the perilymph.

(D) The hair cells form electrical synapses with peripheral regions of bipolar cells.

(E) Deflection of the stereocilia can depolarize the hair cells.

399. All of the following statements concerning hair cells of the utricle are true EXCEPT:

(A) They are stimulated by deformation of their stereocilia by the otolithic membrane.

(B) They are stimulated by angular acceleration of the body.

(C) Deformation of the brush pile of the stereocilia and kinocilium in the direction of the kinocilium opens up many channels, leading to a depolarization.

(D) They are stimulated by tilting of the head or by changing the position of the head.

(E) Deformation of the stereocilia and kinocilium in the direction opposite to that of the kinocilium will result in a hyperpolarization.

400. All of the following concerning the cochlea nuclei are true EXCEPT:

(A) They receive first-order auditory fibers.

(B) They project fibers to the inferior colliculus.

(C) They receive inputs from the opposite ear.

(D) They are tonotopically organized.

(E) The ventral cochlea nucleus projects to the superior olivary nucleus.

401. All of the following statements concerning the auditory cortex are correct EXCEPT:

(A) The auditory cortex is unique in that it contains only a single receiving area for afferent sensory information.

(B) It is functionally organized into columns.

(C) It contains a number of regions which are tonotopically organized.

(D) It receives auditory information from the contralateral temporal cortex via fibers of the corpus callosum.

(E) It contains neurons capable of responding to the presentation of a sequence of tones rather than just a single frequency.

402. All of the following statements concerning the vestibular system are correct EXCEPT:

(A) Vestibular hair cells are innervated by peripheral processes of primary afferent fibers.

(B) Rotation of the head is a sufficient stimulus to activate the maculae of the utricle.

(C) Depolarization of the hair cell occurs when the stereocilia are bent in the direction of the kinocilium.

(D) Primary afferent fibers cease to discharge after rotation of the head ceases.

(E) Vestibular nerve fibers associated with each duct in the semicircular canals are excited by movement in only one direction.

403. All of the following statements concerning the olfactory system are correct EXCEPT:

(A) An olfactory receptor is unique in that it displays little adaptation.

(B) An olfactory stimulus produces a depolarizing receptor potential that leads to an increasing number of action potentials.

(C) The receptor potential occurs when sodium ion channels open.

(D) The capacity of an odorant to increase the discharge rate of olfactory neurons is a function of its ability to stimulate activity of adenylate cyclase.

(E) A single olfactory receptor cell may respond to several different odorants.

404. All of the following statements concerning central functions of vestibular nuclei are correct EXCEPT:

(A) All four vestibular nuclei receive inputs from fibers contained in the vestibular component of cranial nerve VIII.

(B) The lateral vestibular nucleus regulates extensor motor neuron activity.

(C) The medial and superior vestibular nuclei mediate reflex activity involving both vestibular and occulomotor mechanisms.

(D) The inferior vestibular nucleus contributes significantly to the integration of vestibular inputs to the cerebellum.

(E) Vestibular nuclei project axons to the neostriatum for regulation of motor functions.

405. In the olfactory glomerulus, primary afferent fibers terminate principally upon:

(A) granule cell dendrites forming axo-dendritic synapses

(B) granule cell axon terminals forming axo-axonic synapses

(C) mitral cell dendrites forming axo-dendritic synapses

(D) mitral cell axon terminals forming axo-axonic synapses

(E) axon terminals of fibers arising from the olfactory tubercle, forming axo-axonic synapses

406. The part of the olfactory receptor mechanism that initially responds to an olfactory stimulus is:

(A) mitral cell

(B) granule cell

(C) sustentacular cell

(D) basal cell

(E) olfactory cilia

407. The neural basis of olfactory discrimination is believed to utilize:

(A) temporal summation of olfactory signals in the anterior olfactory nucleus

(B) specific activation of different groups of olfactory glomeruli that are spatially organized and segregated within the olfactory bulb

(C) specific activation of different groups of cells within the olfactory tubercle

(D) specific activation of different cell groups within the amygdala

(E) temporal summation of olfactory signals in the mediodorsal thalamic nucleus

408. The principal efferent pathway of the olfactory bulb arises from:

(A) granule cells

(B) Golgi cells

(C) receptor cells

(D) mitral cells

(E) periglomerular cells

409. Direct efferent projections of the olfactory bulb supply:

(A) hypothalamus and prefrontal cortex

(B) amygdala and pyriform cortex

(C) hippocampus and amygdala

(D) prefrontal cortex and medial thalamus

(E) septal area and prefrontal cortex

410. The region of the cortex most closely associated with the conscious perception of smell is:

(A) temporal neocortex

(B) posterior parietal lobule

(C) cingulate gyrus

(D) prefrontal cortex

(E) precentral gyrus

411. Which of the following statements about the taste system is correct:

(A) Receptors for specific taste stimuli are positioned on specific regions of the tongue.

(B) A given taste bud will only respond to a single taste modality.

(C) All taste afferent fibers are contained within the facial nerve.

(D) The cellular mechanism for transduction is essentially the same for each of the categories of taste stimuli.

(E) Single primary taste fibers in the chorda tympani respond to more than one taste stimulus.

412. Which of the following statements concerning "uncinate fits" is correct:

(A) They are characterized by olfactory hallucinations that occur as a result of an irritating lesion of the uncus, adjoining region of the parahippocampal gyrus, or region adjoining the amygdala.

(B) They are characterized by olfactory hallucinations that occur as a result of an irritating lesion of the mediodorsal thalamic nucleus.

(C) They are an epileptic disorder whose focus is the prefrontal cortex and results in a failure to discriminate odors.

(D) They are a partial complex seizure disorder of the amygdala and hippocampus which results in the expression of violent, uncontrolled behavior.

(E) They are an epileptogenic disturbance caused by the formation of a tumor that is limited to the olfactory bulb and which results in a failure to discriminate odors.

413. Which of the following sensory systems is able to utilize a circuit that bypasses the thalamus for the transmission of sensory information from the periphery to the cerebral cortex?

(A) conscious proprioception

(B) taste

(C) olfaction

(D) vision

(E) audition

Sensory Systems

Answers

351-356. The answers are: 351-F, 352-B, 353-E, 354-D, 355-C, 356-A. (Kandel, 3rd Ed., pp. 400-410, 412-415; Guyton, 2nd Ed., pp. 164- 165) The ganglion cells (C) are capable of initiating action potentials (in contrast to the other cells of the retina) and give rise to optic nerve fibers (F) which enter the brain. Bipolar cells (B) serve as interneurons between the photoreceptor cell and the ganglion cell. Horizontal cells (A) also synapse with and are capable of depolarizing receptor cells. Cones (E) are concentrated in the region of the fovea and are associated with day vision, while rods are located throughout the retina and are associated with night vision because their receptive mechanisms are more sensitive to light.

357-363. The answers are: 357-C, 358-E, 359-C, 360-B, 361-E, 362-G, 363-F. (Guyton, 2nd Ed., pp. 144-151) When light rays are focused in front of the retina, myopia (C) results. It can be corrected with a concave lens. In astigmatism (E), the shape of the cornea (and possibly the lens) becomes oblong, resulting in differences in the curvature of the lens along the long and short axes. Accordingly, light is bent differentially with respect to these axes. Astigmatism is corrected with a cylindrical lens. In the condition of hyperopia (B), an individual has a weak lens system and light rays focus behind the retina. It is corrected with a convex lens. Glaucoma (G) is a condition of elevated intraocular pressure caused (perhaps by infection) when debris accumulates in the spaces leading to the canal of Schlemm. If not treated, it can rapidly lead to blindness because the pressure can block conduction along the optic nerve. Cataracts (F) will occur as a result of the denaturing of proteins in the lens fibers. These proteins eventually coagulate, resulting in an opaque lens.

364-369. The answers are: 364-D, 365-F, 366-H, 367-A, 368-C, 369-F. (Kandel, 3rd Ed., pp. 436-438; Carpenter and Sutin, 8th Ed., pp. 542-544) A lesion of the right optic nerve will produce total blindness of the right eye (D) because it damages all of the retinal ganglion cell axons from that eye before any of them can cross at the optic chiasm. A lesion of the right temporal lobe will damage the fibers contained in the loop of Meyer. These are fibers that pass from the lateral geniculate body to the inferior bank of the calcarine sulcus, but they follow a more ventral trajectory which involves parts of the temporal lobe. Accordingly, damage to these fibers will result in an upper left quadrantanopia (F). Since the lower visual fields are represented on the superior bank of the calcarine fissure, a lesion of this region will result in a lower left quadrantanopia (G). A lesion of the right optic tract will damage all of the fibers that are associated with the left visual fields from both eyes.

Accordingly, such a lesion will produce a left homonymous hemianopsia (A). A lesion of the optic chiasm will destroy the crossing fibers associated with the nasal retinal fields. Hence, such a lesion will cause a bitemporal hemianopsia (C).

370. The answer is C. (Kandel, 3rd Ed., pp. 334-337) That sensory systems are somatotopically organized throughout the entirety of their pathways constitutes an essential property of these systems. The somatotopic organization enables an organism to identify the locus of a somatosensory stimulus on the body. If the somatotopic organization did not extend beyond the first synapse, it would be virtually useless and deprive the organism of a critical discriminative capacity. In other systems, such as olfaction, taste, vision, and audition, similar mechanisms are present. For example, in the auditory system, a tonotopic organization is present which enables an organism to discriminate different kinds of frequencies (i.e., tones) and, in the visual system, a retinotopic organization exists which underlies form perception. Sensory systems contain hierarchical organizations which begin at the periphery with the receptor and which then extend to higher order nuclei in the respective pathways involving higher orders of complexity in the processing of sensory information. Parallel processing is also present in sensory systems. This mechanism enables different qualities of a particular stimulus (e.g., the shape and texture of the stimulus) to reach the cortex through different axons along the same pathway. Intensity of a given stimulus is encoded by two properties of neurons: (1) the discharge frequency of a given neuron and (2) the number of neurons activated by a given stimulus. A higher intensity stimulus may cause the neuron to discharge more rapidly and/or cause a greater number of neurons to discharge.

371. The answer is D. (Carpenter and Sutin, 8th Ed., pp. 157-165, 265-270) Meissner's corpuscles, Merkel's discs, and pacinian corpuscles respond to tactile, pressure, or possibly vibratory stimuli, while free nerve endings are associated with nociceptive stimuli. Joint capsules respond to movement of the limb, and the axons of these receptors contribute to the dorsal column-medial lemniscal system mediating the conscious perception of movement.

372. The answer is B. (Kandel, 3rd Ed., pp. 336-338) A rapidly adapting receptor is one that discharges initially to the presence of a stimulus and to any stepwise change in the position or intensity of that stimulus (such as when the stimulus is terminated). A slowly adapting receptor responds continuously (perhaps with a decrease in its frequency) to the presence of the stimulus. A pacinian corpuscle is an example of a rapidly adapting receptor; axons from this receptor contribute to the dorsal column-medial lemniscal system.

373. The answer is E. (Carpenter and Sutin, 8th Ed., pp. 162-164; Kandel, 3rd Ed., pp. 344-346) Meissner's corpuscles differ from pacinian corpuscles in a number of ways. Meissner's corpuscles have smaller receptive fields and can resolve finer spatial differences than can pacinian corpuscles. Meissner's corpuscles are more sensitive to low frequency mechanical stimuli; pacinian corpuscles are more sensitive to high frequency stimuli. In addition, while both receptors are encapsulated, the pacinian corpuscle has a much more well developed perineural capsule than does Meissner's corpuscle. However, because Meissner's corpuscle is coupled to adjoining tissue by connective tissue, it behaves like pacinian corpuscles in the presence of a stimulus — namely, they are both rapidly adapting receptors.

374. The answer is D. (Kandel, 3rd Ed., pp. 368-370) To generate an excitatory focus with an inhibitory surround, three types of inhibition are present in the dorsal column nuclei. First-order neurons ascending in the dorsal columns makes synaptic contact with different cells in the dorsal column nuclei and excite those cells. One such cell may be an inhibitory interneuron that makes synaptic contact with a neighboring dorsal column nuclear cell, thus, inhibiting that cell (i.e., feed forward inhibition). In addition, the dorsal column cell that is excited by the first-order neuron may make synaptic contact with another inhibitory interneuron (in addition to its classical ascending projection to the ventral posterolateral nucleus (VPL) of the thalamus). This inhibitory interneuron makes synaptic contact with an adjacent dorsal column cell and inhibits that cell (i.e., feedback inhibition). Finally, a descending fiber from the postcentral gyrus can make synaptic contact with inhibitory interneurons that inhibit dorsal column cells. The figure below illustrates feedback, feed forward, and descending inhibition. Inhibitory neurons are depicted in black.

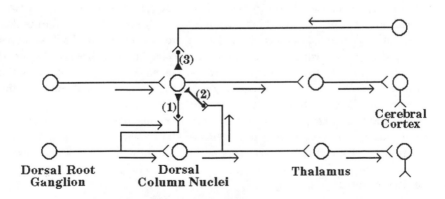

(1) **Feed-Forward Inhibition**
(2) **Feed-Back Inhibition**
(3) **Descending Inhibition**

375. The answer is B. (Carpenter and Sutin, 8th Ed., pp. 265-270; Kandel, 3rd Ed., pp. 334-365; Guyton, 2nd Ed., pp. 104-106) Pacinian corpuscles are examples of rapidly adapting receptors. The characteristic feature of these receptors is they respond when the stimulus is first applied and when it is terminated but not during the intervening period of stimulation. The reason for this property apparently relates to their structural arrangement. The Pacinian corpuscle is an encapsulated receptor that is composed of viscoelastic concentric layers of connective tissue. When a force is applied to one side of the receptor, it is transmitted via the viscous component to its central core, producing a receptor potential. There is a rapid redistribution of the fluid in the capsule which equalizes pressure throughout the receptor. This results in a cessation of the receptor potential within several hundred milliseconds following the onset of the stimulus. All of the other statements presented in this question are correct. The way in which a stimulus is perceived is a function of the way in which the receptor responds to that stimulus. A slowly adapting or rapidly adapting receptor will respond to different qualities of a stimulus. As the stimulus intensity is increased, the rate of discharge of the receptor will also increase. A tonic pressure receptor is one whose discharge rate remains relatively constant in the presence of the stimulus. Ascending fibers within the dorsal column-medial lemniscal pathway display parallel processing of sensory information. For example, some neurons within this pathway convey information about the texture of an object to the postcentral gyrus while others convey information concerning shape. Each of these neuronal groups are activated by mechanoreceptors located in different regions of the hand.

376. The answer is D. (Kandel, 3rd Ed., pp. 374-377) Where two-point discrimination involves small distances between stimuli, an important factor is the presence of large numbers of receptors in the area, producing receptive fields that correspond to discrete, relatively small areas of the body surface. The distance for making two-point discrimination in a given body region is inversely proportional to the number of receptors present. However, other factors are also involved. Each stimulus generates a zone of central excitation that is reflected through all relay stations of the sensory pathway and that provides an important physiological substrate for the phenomenon. Moreover, the separate zones of excitation are enhanced by the mechanism of lateral inhibition. Here, weaker zones of excitation generated from each of these stimuli are eliminated by the inhibitory mechanism (i.e., feed forward and feedback inhibition). This process sharpens the two peaks of excitation which enhances the distinction between them. All inhibition within the somatosensory system occurs within the central nervous system, not peripherally where the receptor is located.

377. The answer is E. (Kandel, 3rd Ed., pp. 378-381) As a general rule, neurons situated in the cortex in association with any of the sensory systems take on a much higher level of complexity than neurons situated at lower levels of the relay network. In the case of the somatosensory system, direction-sensitive cells in the somatosensory cortex will respond to one direction of movement of a stimulus along the receptive field and not to another direction. Orientation-sensitive neurons respond best to movement along one axis of the receptive field. This is not true for neurons situated in lower levels of the somatosensory pathway.

378. The answer is A. (Kandel, 3rd Ed., pp. 385-398) Substance P is the transmitter (or neuromodulator) released at primary afferent terminals of the pain pathway within the substantia gelatinosa. Opiate receptors are present at the primary afferent terminals in the spinal cord of the pain pathway and are involved in the presynaptic and postsynaptic inhibitory actions at those sites. They are presumably also present at medullary levels where descending opioidergic fibers from the midbrain periaqueductal gray synapse. However, there is no evidence that the lateral hypothalamus plays any role in the modulation of pain.

379. The answer is B. (Kandel, 3rd Ed., pp. 385-387) Most of the substances noted in this question have the capacity of activating primary pain afferent fibers. For example, potassium and histamine are released from damaged cells in response to injury and excite the primary pain afferents. Prostaglandins, metabolites of arachidonic acid, produce hyperalgesia after being released from damaged cells. Bradykinin is also released as a result of tissue damage and is an active pain-producing substance. It causes the release of prostaglandins from neighboring cells and activates the primary afferent pain fibers. On the other hand, enkephalins block pain conduction at the first synapse located in the dorsal horn of the spinal cord.

380. The answer is C. (Kandel, 3rd Ed., pp. 388-389) Referred pain is a phenomenon in which pain impulses, arising from primary afferent fibers from one part of the body (such as from deep visceral structures), terminate on dorsal horn projection neurons that normally receive cutaneous afferents from a different part of the body (such as the arm). In this situation, an individual who might be suffering a heart attack experiences pain that appears to be coming from the arm. It is the convergence of these distinctly different inputs onto the same projection neurons which provide the basis for this phenomenon. None of the other possible mechanisms that are listed in this question are considered viable possibilities since they have no anatomical or physiological basis.

381. The answer is D. (Kandel, 3rd Ed., pp. 389-390)   Primary nociceptive afferent fibers would have to release an excitatory transmitter in order for normal transmission to take place.   Two excitatory transmitters have been identified in association with different classes of primary nociceptive afferents: substance P and excitatory amino acids. The best candidate as an excitatory amino acid is glutamate. Since enkephalins have been shown to be inhibitory transmitters in the pain system, they are not likely to be released from the primary afferents. Instead, other central nervous system neurons impinge upon the primary afferents and enkephalins are released from those neurons.

382. The answer is E. (Kandel, 3rd Ed., pp. 390-392)   Ascending fibers associated with nociception make synaptic contact with a number of nuclear groups at different levels of the neuraxis.   These nuclear groups include the lateral cervical nucleus of the dorsal horn of the spinal cord, medullary reticular formation, midbrain periaqueductal gray, and the ventral posterolateral nucleus (VPL) of the thalamus.   All of these structures have been implicated in the transmission or modulation of pain impulses. Pain inputs from the region of the head are distributed to the spinal trigeminal nucleus rather than the main sensory nucleus of nerve V.

383. The answer is B. (Kandel, 3rd Ed., pp. 392-394)   Perhaps, one of the most important discoveries in pain research made over the past 15 years is of a descending pathway, originating in the midbrain periaqueductal gray and making synaptic contacts in the medulla.   From the medulla this pathway descends to the dorsal horn where these fibers provide the anatomical substrate for suppression of pain inputs that enter the spinal cord from the periphery. There are no known inputs to the cortex that directly produce analgesia.   The mechanism governing analgesia appears to operate at lower brainstem and spinal cord levels. The classical ascending fibers for transmission of pain impulses reach thalamic nuclei directly and, thus, local interneurons within the midbrain would not be able to interfere with such transmission. The pathway to the ventral posterolateral nucleus (VPL) of the thalamus is an excitatory one and is not known to have any inhibitory properties.   Cholinergic neurons in the basal forebrain have been implicated in memory functions and are not known to have any role in the regulation of pain sensation.

384. The answer is B. (Kandel, 3rd Ed., pp. 393-394)   The classical descending pathway for central inhibition of nociception involves the following pathway: fibers that originate in the midbrain periaqueductal gray matter project caudally to the level of the nucleus raphe magnus upon whose neurons they synapse. Fibers from the nucleus raphe magnus then project further caudally where they synapse in the dorsal horn of the spinal cord.

385. The answer is B. (Kandel, 3rd Ed., pp. 420-428) The lateral geniculate is a classical sensory relay nucleus of the thalamus. It receives a visuotopic projection from the retina whereby fibers from the contralateral retina terminate on cells that are different from the ones that receive ipsilateral retinal afferents. Lateral geniculate cell axons project to the primary visual cortex (i.e., area 17 and not area 19) and, in turn, the lateral geniculate nucleus receives reciprocal connections from the visual cortex. The physiological properties of the geniculate bear a resemblance to those of the retina, especially since both contain cells with circular symmetrical receptive fields.

386. The answer is C. (Kandel, 3rd Ed. pp. 396-397) Evidence indicates that within the dorsal horn of the spinal cord, descending pain inhibitory fibers from the lower brainstem (serotonergic and noradrenergic fibers) synapse upon interneurons that are enkephalinergic. These enkephalinergic neurons then synapse upon both presynaptic terminals of primary pain afferent fibers as well as upon the dendrites of dorsal horn projection neurons (which also receive inputs from the primary nociceptive afferent fibers).

387. The answer is B. (Kandel, 3rd Ed., pp. 402-405) The major functional difference between rods and cones is that rods by being more sensitive to light than cones are specialized for night vision. Cones are specialized for day (and color) vision. The visual pigments contained in the outer segments capture light which results in a change in ionic fluxes across the plasma membrane of the photoreceptor cell. These ionic fluxes ultimately lead to action potentials in retinal ganglion cells. Finally, the signal is conducted to the lateral geniculate body via fibers of the optic nerve and optic tract.

388. The answer is A. (Kandel, 3rd Ed., pp. 403-408; Guyton, 2nd Ed., pp. 155-157) In the presence of light, rhodopsin, found in the outer segment of the rod, breaks down. The breakdown products of rhodopsin include a series of unstable intermediate molecules, including metarhodopsin II, which then further breaks down into scotopsin and all-trans retinal. In the reformation of rhodopsin, all-trans retinal is then isomerized into 11-cis retinal, which combines with scotopsin to reform rhodopsin. All of the other statements in this question are correct. The rod cell is unique among sensory receptors in that it is hyperpolarized in the presence of the sensory stimulus to which it responds. The hyperpolarization of the cell in darkness is the result of an inward flow of sodium ions. However, in the presence of light, metarhodopsin II, formed from the breakdown of rhodopsin, activates the protein, transducin, which, in turn, activates larger numbers of phosphodiesterase molecules. Phosphodiesterase catalyzes the hydrolysis of cyclic GMP molecules. Because sodium ions utilize "cyclic GMP channels" to enter the cell, these channels become closed in the presence of light. With the breakdown of metarhodopsin II, there is a reversal of this process to the condition where sodium channels are open.

389. The answer is C. (Kandel, 3rd Ed., pp. 410-430) Both retina ganglion cells and lateral geniculate neurons exhibit an "on-center" and "off-surround" with respect to objects in the receptive field. Cells in area 18 of the visual cortex are not known to possess these characteristics. Cells in layer 4 of the primary visual cortex do not have circular receptive fields. Instead, these cells respond to such stimuli as lines and bars.

390. The answer is A. (Kandel, 3rd Ed., pp. 413-415) When a cone is hyperpolarized by light there is a reduction in the release of transmitter substance (glutamate). This reduced amount of transmitter results in excitation of the "on-center" bipolar cell and inhibition of the "off-center" bipolar cell (presumably because the two types of bipolar cell contain different postsynaptic receptors). Since bipolar cells excite the ganglion cells, an "off-center" bipolar cell will be inhibited when light is present and, thus, will be unable to excite the ganglion cell to which it is connected. "On-center" bipolar cells are excited when light is present and so are the ganglion cells to which they are connected. In addition, "on-center" bipolar cells inhibit ganglion cells that receive their primary input from "off-center" bipolar cells. This serves to increase the likelihood that these ganglion cells will remain inhibited when the light stimulus is present. A cone cell may make synaptic contact with two types of bipolar cells ("on-center" or "off-center"). Because they possess different postsynaptic receptor mechanisms, the two types of bipolar cells will respond differently to input from cones.

391. The answer is D. (Guyton, 2nd Ed., pp. 157-168) Fibers of the optic tract synapse in a number of regions associated with the processing of visual information or visual reflex activity. These include the lateral geniculate nuclei (part of the classical visual pathway for relaying visual information to the visual cortex), the pretectal area (for elicitation of the pupillary light reflex and reflex movements of the eyes), the superior colliculus (for bilateral control of rapid eye movements), and the suprachiasmatic nucleus (which relates to the control of circadian rhythms). There are no known monosynaptic projections from the retina to the nuclei of cranial nerves III and IV.

392. The answer is E. (Kandel, 3rd Ed., pp. 409-415) Lateral inhibition within the retina is generated most effectively by the horizontal cells. A horizontal cell receives inputs from a given receptor cell and, when activated, inhibits adjacent receptor cells. It is possible for a given cone cell to differentially affect two neighboring bipolar cells and for an "on-center" bipolar cell to hyperpolarize an adjacent "off- center" ganglion cell. However, the primary flow of information through these neuronal elements is in the plane of orientation that most directly connects the receptor cell to the ganglion cell through a bipolar cell. Therefore, the contribution of these elements to lateral inhibition is relatively minimal (if at all) in comparison to the effects generated by horizontal cells. The ganglion cell is not known to play any role in lateral inhibition.

393. The answer is B. (Guyton, 2nd Ed., pp. 164-169) Half of the fibers of the optic tract project to the lateral geniculate nucleus of a given side. The temporal fibers, which are uncrossed, project to layers II, III, and V, while the nasal retinal fibers, which are crossed, pass to layers I, IV, and VI. In addition, layers I and II are unique in that they contain large cells that receive inputs from Y ganglion cells. These are the largest of the ganglion cells and are important for the transmission of instantaneous changes in the visual image to the visual cortex. Moreover, these retinal inputs can be "gated" (modulated) by virtue of descending cortical fibers from the ipsilateral primary visual cortex.

394. The answer is E. (Guyton, 2nd Ed., pp. 167-168) Layers III-VI of the dorsolateral geniculate nucleus contain cells that are considerably smaller in size than those found in layers I and II. The important feature of this region is it receives inputs from the most numerous of the retinal ganglion cells (X cells) which transmit information about color vision and provide a very accurate, point-to-point, transmission to the visual cortex. The lateral geniculate nucleus does not receive any inputs from the hypothalamus.

395. The answer is C. (Kandel, 3rd Ed., pp. 431-434, 473-474; Guyton, 2nd Ed., pp. 168-170) Many cells of the visual cortex project their axons to neighboring as well as distant regions of the brain. However, those of the deepest part of layer 4 (layer 4c), which mainly receives afferent impulses, make, at best, only local connections. It should be noted that the visual cortex, like other regions of cortex, has a columnar organization that can be functionally divided. For example, a given column may be an orientation column (i.e., contains cells that respond to light bars with specific axes of orientation). The visual cortex also contains columns that receive information from either the right or left eye and are thus called ocular dominance columns. Blob zones are present within ocular dominance columns which are dedicated to the analysis of color and which have receptive fields that have no specific orientation.

396. The answer is B. (Kandel, 3rd Ed., pp. 467-477; Guyton, 2nd Ed., pp. 157-159) The classical theories of color vision assume the existence of three types of photoreceptors that are selectively responsive to light of red, green, or blue wavelengths. Retinal ganglion cells and lateral geniculate neurons both display concentric, single opponent properties. This means that they respond maximally to a stimulus of a given wavelength (e.g., green) presented in the center of their receptive field and are inhibited when an opponent wavelength (e.g., red) is presented. It is important to note that each of these cells possesses a center-surround receptive field organization. Under these conditions, a spot of white light applied to the center of the receptive field will cause the cell to discharge, while the same light presented to the surround will cause it to be inhibited. Moreover, with respect to specific single-opponent cells, the center-surround organization may function as follows: if the center of the receptive field is maximally activated by a green wavelength, which produces a maximal discharge of the neuron, the surround may be activated by cones sensitive to a red wavelength. Concentric double-opponent cells are found in blobs in the visual cortex and respond maximally to contrasts of red-green or yellow-blue.

397. The answer is C. (Kandel, 3rd Ed., pp. 426-431; Guyton, 2nd Ed., pp. 169-171) Cells in the lateral geniculate nucleus respond very much like ganglion cells in the retina because of the point-to-point projection pathway from the retina to the lateral geniculate. Accordingly, lateral geniculate cells have small concentric receptive fields that are either on-center or off-center in which the cells respond best to small spots of light that are in the center of the receptive field. On the other hand, cells in the visual cortex display a much greater complexity in their responses to images in the visual field. Instead of responding to small spots of light, they respond to lines and borders in the different areas of the visual field. In particular, the simple cell responds as a function of the retinal position in which the line-stimulus is located as well as its orientation (e.g., whether it is in a vertical or horizontal position). As a result, when a bar of light is positioned in the appropriate part of the visual field with the appropriate orientation, the cells in area 17 will respond maximally. When either of these parameters is altered, the firing pattern of the cell will be reduced or totally inhibited. Complex cells lack clear excitatory and inhibitory zones (i.e., these neurons respond to bars of light in a given orientation but they are not position specific). Other cells, called hypercomplex cells, are stimulated by bars of light of specific lengths, or by specific shapes.

398. The answer is D. (Kandel, 3rd Ed., pp. 482-489; Guyton, 2nd Ed., pp. 178-182) The peripheral regions of bipolar cells forming the spiral ganglion make synaptic contact with the hair cells. This is a chemical synapse. However, the transmitter has yet to be identified. All of the question's other choices are correct. Different regions of the basilar membrane are sensitive to different frequencies of sound. High frequencies cause the membrane to vibrate maximally at its base, while low frequencies cause it to vibrate maximally at the apex. The stereocilia of hair cells are attached to the tectorial membrane. As a result of vibration caused by sound, the basilar membrane moves up and down, resulting in a shearing movement of the hair cells against the tectorial membrane. It is the physical bending of the hair cells toward the scala vestibuli that causes them to depolarize. There is also an activation of voltage-gated calcium channels that further amplifies the depolarization of the hair cells. Movement of the hair cells in the opposite direction will produce hyperpolarization. Since there is a marked difference between the ion concentration in the endolymph of the scala media and that in the perilymph of the scala tympani and scala vestibuli, a potential of +80 mV exists between the endolymph and perilymph. This potential is called the endocochlear potential.

399. The answer is B. (Kandel, 3rd Ed., pp. 503-506; Guyton, 2nd Ed., pp. 218-219) Very fine filaments connect the tip of each stereocilia to the next and these cilia project upward into the gelatinous layer in which calcium carbonate crystals (i.e., statoconia) are embedded. When the head is suddenly tilted or the position of the head is suddenly changed, the statoconia, which have greater inertia than the surrounding fluids, are moved backward onto the cilia. Deflection of the stereocilia in the direction of the kinocilium causes an opening of channels for conducting sodium ions. Hyperpolarization occurs when the stereocilia are bent in the direction opposite to that of the kinocilium, in which case, tension on the attachments is reduced, which results in the closing of sodium channels. Hair cells of the utricle are not stimulated by angular acceleration. This type of stimulus is effective, however, in activating receptors in the semicircular canals.

400. The answer is C. (Kandel, 3rd Ed., pp. 491-494; Guyton, 2nd Ed., pp. 183-184) The dorsal cochlea nucleus receives first-order eighth cranial nerve fibers associated with audition and projects its neurons to the inferior colliculus, contralaterally, and to the superior olivary nucleus, bilaterally. The dorsal cochlea nucleus is tonotopically organized in that cells in one region respond preferentially to a given frequency while cells in other regions of this nucleus respond preferentially to other frequencies. The dorsal cochlea nucleus does not receive inputs from the contralateral ear.

401. The answer is A. (Kandel, 3rd Ed., pp. 483-486; Guyton, 2nd Ed., pp. 184-185; Carpenter and Sutin, 8th Ed., p. 679) Similar to other regions of cortex, the auditory cortex also maintains a columnar organization. Within the auditory cortex, there are a number of regions that display a tonotopic organization. However, many of the cells of the auditory cortex have the unique capacity to respond to a series of frequencies presented together (i.e., sequential pattern of sounds). This represents a more complex response than for cells in lower levels of the auditory pathway. This is strikingly similar to the complexity observed in the visual cortex in which cells respond to a line and its orientation rather than just to a spot of light. The auditory cortex also receives inputs from the contralateral auditory cortex by way of the corpus callosum. Such inputs may serve to aid in detecting the direction from which a sound arises. Similar to other sensory areas of the cortex, there are multiple regions which receive auditory signals. These regions surround the primary auditory receiving area but are also situated in the temporal lobe.

402. The answer is B. (Kandel, 3rd Ed., pp. 504-507; Guyton 2nd Ed., pp. 217-220) Rotation of the head, called angular acceleration, is a sufficient stimulus to activate the receptors contained in the semicircular canals. It is not a sufficient stimulus for the maculae of the utricle, which requires linear acceleration. The other choices of the question are correct. Hair cells make synaptic contact with peripheral processes of primary afferent fibers and, thus, action potentials can be evoked in these primary afferents as a result of the depolarization of the hair cells. When the stereocilia are bent in the direction of the kinocilium as a result of rotation in a given direction (which is caused by the movement of endolymph in one direction), depolarization occurs because this bending results in the opening of channels which allow sodium ions to flow into the cell (causing depolarization). When the rotation ceases, the endolymph continues to rotate but the turning of the semicircular ducts has ceased, thus causing the hair cells to be moved in the opposite direction. It is the movement of the stereocilia in the opposite direction that now produces hyperpolarization of the hair cell because sodium channels close. Since the semicircular canals are arranged in different planes (i.e., anterior and posterior vertical canals and a horizontal canal), primary afferent fibers associated with each of these canals will respond to movement in only one direction.

403. The answer is A. (Kandel, 3rd Ed., pp. 513-516; Guyton, 2nd Ed., pp. 191-192) An olfactory receptor shows a rapid adaptation (approximately 50%) during the first few seconds and little adaptation afterwards. Within the olfactory system, an olfactory stimulus opens sodium channels producing depolarizing receptor potentials that lead to action potentials. The action potentials increase in frequency to about 20/s. It has also been shown that the discharge rate of olfactory neurons is a function of the degree to which adenylate cyclase activity is stimulated. Adenylate cyclase catalyzes the formation of cyclic AMP, which, in turn, causes the opening of many additional channels. There probably exists a large number of olfactory receptors and each one most likely is capable of recognizing several different odorants (as determined by electrophysiological experiments).

404. The answer is E. (Kandel, 3rd Ed., pp. 508-510) All four vestibular nuclei receive inputs from the vestibular branch of cranial nerve VIII. The lateral vestibular nucleus projects to all levels of the spinal cord and provides powerful excitation of both alpha and gamma extensor motor neurons. Thus, as a result of this mechanism, the lateral vestibular nucleus can influence postural mechanisms. The superior and medial nuclei project their axons rostrally through the medial longitudinal fasciculus to cranial nerve nuclei (III, IV, and VI) that innervate the extraocular eye muscles. In addition, the medial nucleus projects fibers to the cervical cord where they synapse with motor neurons that innervate neck muscles. In this manner, these nuclei serve to integrate signals that affect these nuclei and allow for simultaneous rotation of the eyes in a direction opposite that in which the head is tilted. The inferior (and medial) nuclei also project to the cerebellum. The inferior vestibular nucleus also receives inputs from the cerebellar vermis. In so doing, this nucleus appears to integrate information linked to the vestibular apparatus and parts of the cerebellum. Although there is some evidence that secondary vestibular fibers project to thalamic relay nuclei such as ventral posterolateral (VPL), there is no evidence that vestibular fibers project to any region of the neostriatum (or basal ganglia as a whole for that matter).

405. The answer is C. (Kandel, 3rd Ed., pp. 515-417; Carpenter and Sutin, 8th Ed., pp. 614-615; Guyton, 2nd Ed., pp. 191-193) The olfactory receptor and its primary afferent fiber terminate upon dendrites of mitral cells. This relationship is of importance because it is the axon of the mitral cell that projects out of the olfactory bulb (forming the major component of the lateral olfactory stria). The granule cell processes make synaptic contact with dendrites of mitral cells, forming dendro-dendritic synapses, but are not known to make synaptic contact with primary afferent terminals. Cells arising in the olfactory tubercle are not known to project to the olfactory bulb. Instead, projections of cells situated in the olfactory tubercle contribute fibers to the medial forebrain bundle and stria medullaris.

406. The answer is E. (Kandel, 3rd Ed., pp. 312-314; Guyton, 2nd Ed., pp. 191-192) The olfactory cilia are extensions of the receptor cell and it is this part of the cell that initially responds to an olfactory stimulus. The cilia contain protein membranes that bind with different odorants which constitutes a necessary condition for excitation of the olfactory cell. Mitral and granule cells are situated in the olfactory bulb and, consequently, are not part of the receptor mechanism. Sustentacular cells are supporting cells and are not part of the receptor mechanism. Basal cells are the precursor cells for receptor cells and, thus, are also not directly part of the receptor mechanism.

407. The answer is B. (Kandel, 3rd Ed., pp. 516-518; Guyton, 2nd Ed., p. 193) A number of recent studies have indicated that different olfactory glomeruli respond to different kinds of olfactory stimuli. In a sense this represents a type of organization of the olfactory bulb that bears a functional similarity to the spatial organization that exists for other sensory systems. There is no evidence that such a spatial arrangement exists for other components of the olfactory system, nor is there any evidence that temporal summation plays any role in the process of olfactory discrimination.

408. The answer is D. (Carpenter and Sutin, 8th Ed., pp. 613-616) The principal output pathways of the olfactory bulb arise from mitral cells and a related cell called tufted cells. The mitral cells project their axons out of the olfactory bulb to other regions of the forebrain associated with the transmission of olfactory information to the cerebral cortex. The major pathway subserving this is the lateral olfactory stria. Other cells that are mentioned in this question are either not present in the olfactory bulb (i.e., Golgi cells) or they have no known projections outside of the olfactory bulb. Receptor cells project only as far as the glomerulus. The granule cell has no axon. The periglomerular cell makes only local connections among neighboring glomeruli.

409. The answer is B. (Carpenter and Sutin, 8th Ed., pp. 615-618; Kandel, 3rd Ed., p. 518) Mitral cell axons enter the lateral olfactory stria and project caudally through this bundle to supply the medial amygdala and pyriform cortex. Olfactory projections to other nuclei such as the hippocampal formation, prefrontal cortex, medial thalamus and septal area require at least one additional synaptic connection such as in the pyriform cortex, amygdala, or olfactory tubercle.

410. The answer is D. (Kandel, 3rd Ed., pp. 517-518) Experimental evidence indicates the prefrontal cortex is a key region for the conscious perception of smell. This conclusion is based upon: (1) the prefrontal cortex receives major inputs from the olfactory bulb by the following routes: olfactory bulb —> pyriform cortex —> prefrontal cortex, or olfactory bulb —> pyriform cortex (and olfactory tubercle) —> mediodorsal thalamic nucleus —> prefrontal cortex, and (2) lesions of the prefrontal cortex result in a failure to discriminate odors. Olfactory functions are not known to be associated with any of the other choices. Instead, the primary auditory receiving area is located in the auditory cortex; the posterior parietal lobule is concerned with such processes as the programming mechanisms associated with complex motor tasks; the cingulate gyrus has been associated with such functions as spatial learning and the modulation of autonomic and emotional processes; and the prefrontal gyrus contains the primary motor area.

411. The answer is E. (Kandel, 3rd Ed., pp. 521-525) A primary afferent fiber innervates many taste receptors. Recordings from the primary afferent fiber reveal that it responds to different modalities of taste stimuli, although it may preferentially respond to a single, given modality. This would suggest that taste discrimination and perception occur as a result of the comparison of the activation pattern of different groups of taste fibers. Different types of taste receptors may be positioned in the same region of the tongue. Primary afferent taste fibers respond to more than one modality of taste stimuli. Taste fibers from the anterior two-thirds of the tongue are carried in the facial nerve; fibers from the posterior third of the tongue are carried in the glossopharyngeal nerve, and taste fibers from the epiglottis are carried in the vagus nerve. The cellular mechanism for transduction of taste stimuli depends upon the stimulus. For example, receptors for molecules associated with sweet and bitter tastes utilize second messengers, while those associated with sour and salty tasting molecules act directly upon the ion channels.

412. The answer is A. (Kandel, 3rd Ed., p. 518; Carpenter and Sutin, 8th Ed., p. 621) Uncinate fits are characterized by seizure activity involving portions of the anterior aspect of the temporal lobe. The structures most often implicated include the uncus, parahippocampal gyrus, the region of the amygdala and adjoining tissue, and the pyriform cortex. During the occurrence of uncinate fits, individuals experience olfactory hallucinations of a highly unpleasant nature.

413. The answer is C. (Carpenter and Sutin, 8th Ed., pp. 266, 344-345, 372, 541, 613-617) The pathway for conscious proprioception from the body utilizes the ventral posterolateral nucleus as its thalamic relay. Conscious proprioception from the head utilizes the ventral posteromedial nucleus (VPM) as its relay. The taste pathway utilizes VPM as well. The visual system utilizes the lateral geniculate nucleus, and the auditory system utilizes the medial geniculate nucleus. In contrast, the olfactory system can transmit olfactory information to the prefrontal cortex without engaging thalamic nuclei. Thus, olfactory information reaches the pyriform cortex and amygdala from the olfactory bulb and then is transmitted directly to the prefrontal cortex. However, it should be noted that olfactory information also can reach the prefrontal cortex by virtue of projections from the olfactory tubercle and pyriform cortex via the mediodorsal thalamic nucleus. Thus, the olfactory system may utilize a parallel processing mechanism in transmitting inputs to the prefrontal cortex.

Forebrain Anatomy

DIRECTIONS: The questions below consist of lettered headings followed by a set of numbered items. For each numbered item select the **one** point on the figure with which it is **most** closely associated. Each lettered heading may be used **once, more than once, or not at all.**

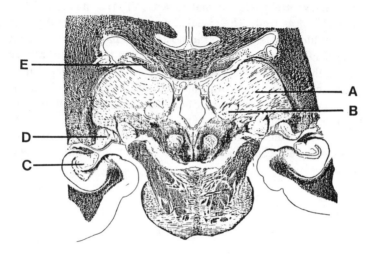

(Adapted from Villiger, Fig. 27; with permission.)

Questions 414-418 Refer to the figure above.

414. neurons in this region project their axons to the inferior parietal lobule

415. this fiber bundle arises from the hippocampal formation

416. a lesion of this structure produces short-term memory deficits

417. a specific relay nucleus

418. neurons in this region innervate the striatum

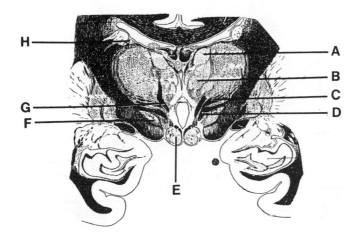

(Adapted from Villiger, Fig. 34; with permission.)

Questions 419-426 Refer to the figure above.

419. fibers contained in this bundle arise from both cerebellum and basal ganglia

420. maintains reciprocal connections with the globus pallidus

421. receives fibers from the mammillary bodies and projects axons to the cingulate gyrus

422. contains a major efferent pathway of the basomedial amygdala

427. these fibers arise from the dorsal aspect of the medial pallidal segment

424. axons arising from this region project to the anterior thalamic nucleus

425. these fibers arise from the mammillary bodies

426. axons arising from this region supply large parts of the frontal lobe

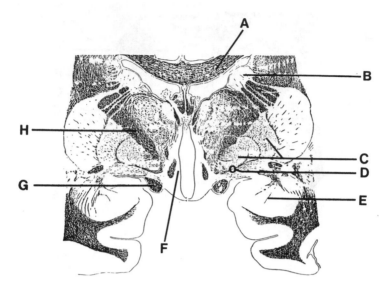

(Adapted from Villiger, Fig. 38; with permission.)

Questions 427-433 Refer to the figure above.

427. these fibers arise from deeper cortical layers (layers V-VI)

428. these fibers arise from more superficial layers (layers II-IV) of the cerebral cortex

429. this region contains the cell bodies of origin of fibers which constitute the major efferent pathway of the basal ganglia

430. this structure receives a significant dopaminergic input from the substantia nigra

431. cells in this region produce vasopressin and oxytocin

432. major afferent source of the hypothalamus

433. these fibers specifically supply the ventrolateral (VL), ventral anterior (VA), and centromedian (CM) thalamic nuclei

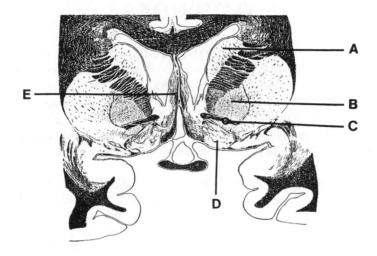

(Adapted from Villiger, Fig. 44; with permission.)

Questions 434-438 Refer to the figure above.

434. this structure receives afferent fibers from the cerebral cortex and thalamus

435. this structure is the source of a major cholinergic projection to the neocortex

436. this structure receives inputs from the neostriatum

437. this structure transmits olfactory information from the anterior olfactory nucleus

438. this structure (which is considerably larger in nonhumans such as rat, cat, and monkey) is a component of the limbic system and receives a major afferent projection from the hippocampal formation

Forebrain Anatomy

Answers

414-418. The answers are: 414-A, 415-E, 416-C, 417-D, 418-B. (Carpenter and Sutin, 8th Ed., pp. 493-534, 579-604, 618-623) This section is taken at the level of the posterior thalamus and, because of the oblique cut, also includes parts of the midbrain and pons. The fornix (E), situated just below the corpus callosum, arises from the hippocampal formation and supplies the septal area, anterior thalamic nucleus, and the mammillary bodies. The hippocampal formation (C) is associated with a number of different processes including short-term memory. Thus, a lesion of this structure will likely produce deficits in short-term memory. The lateral geniculate nucleus (D), situated in the far ventrolateral aspect of the posterior thalamus, is a classical relay nucleus for the transmission of visual information to the cortex. The centromedian nucleus (B), identified by its encapsulated appearance, can be found in posterior levels of the thalamus where it projects to the neostriatum. Also located at the level of the posterior aspect of the thalamus is the pulvinar nucleus (A). This large structure projects its axons to the inferior parietal lobule.

419-426. The answers are: 419-D, 420-F, 421-A, 422-H, 423-C, 424-E, 425-G, 426-B. (Carpenter and Sutin, 8th Ed., pp. 493-534, 579-604, 618-638) This section is taken at the level of the mammillary bodies (at ventral levels) and includes parts of the anterior thalamus (at dorsal levels). The subthalamic nucleus (F), which lies on the dorsal surface of the internal capsule, maintains reciprocal connections with the globus pallidus through a pathway called the subthalamic fasciculus. The anterior nucleus of the thalamus (A), which lies at the rostral end of the thalamus in a dorsomedial position, receives a major input from the mammillary bodies via the mammillothalamic tract. Fibers arising from the anterior nucleus supply the cingulate cortex. The region immediately below the tail and body of the caudate nucleus is occupied by a major output pathway of the basomedial amygdala called the stria terminalis (H). It supplies the medial preoptic region, bed nucleus of the stria terminalis, and medial hypothalamus. The thalamic fasciculus (C) can be seen in sections taken through the caudal half of the thalamus and is clearly visualized in a position dorsal to the subthalamic nucleus and lenticular fasciculus. It contains fibers that arise from both the dentate nucleus of the cerebellum and the medial pallidal segment. The mammillary bodies (E), situated at the base of the posterior aspect of hypothalamus, are the origin of the mammillothalamic tract (G) which innervates the anterior thalamic nucleus. A large nuclear mass situated in the medial aspect of the posterior two-thirds of the thalamus is the mediodorsal nucleus (B). Its cortically directed fibers supply much of the frontal lobe, including the prefrontal cortex. The lenticular fasciculus (D), situated just below the thalamic fasciculus and immediately above the subthalamic nucleus at the level of this brain section, arises from the dorsomedial aspect of the medial pallidal segment and supplies several thalamic nuclei.

427-433. The answers are: 427-H, 428-A, 429-C, 430-B, 431-F, 432-E, 433-D. (Carpenter and Sutin, 8th Ed., pp. 493-534, 579-604, 618-638, 646-648) This section is taken from rostral levels of the diencephalon. Fibers of the corpus callosum (A) arise from more superficial layers of the cortex (layers II-IV) and project to the homotypic region of the contralateral cortex. The globus pallidus (C) constitutes the major source of efferent fibers of the basal ganglia. The caudate nucleus (B) receives dopaminergic inputs from the substantia nigra. Different cells in the paraventricular nucleus of hypothalamus (F), situated in the dorsomedial region at anterior levels, synthesize oxytocin and vasopressin. These hormones are transported down their axons to the posterior pituitary. Different fiber groups of the amygdala (E) provide major inputs into the medial and lateral regions of the hypothalamus and thus constitute a significant modulator of hypothalamic functions. Fibers of the ansa lenticularis (D) arise from the ventral aspect of the medial pallidal segment and can be visualized at more anterior levels of the pallidum. Its axons supply the ventrolateral (VL), ventral anterior (VA), and centromedian (CM) nuclei of the thalamus. Corticobulbar and corticospinal fibers contained within the internal capsule (H) arise from deeper layers (layers V-VI) of the frontal and parietal lobes.

434-438. The answers are: 434-A, 435-D, 436-B, 437-C, 438-E. (Carpenter and Sutin, 8th Ed., pp. 579-632) This section is taken at the level of the septum pellucidum, anterior commissure, and the substantia innominata. Fibers from the region of the basal nucleus of Meynert located in the substantia innominata (D) (at the base of the brain in the far rostral forebrain) send a cholinergic projection to wide areas of the neocortex. The globus pallidus (B) receives inputs from the neostriatum (i.e., caudate nucleus and putamen). The anterior commissure (C) can be clearly seen at the level of the forebrain just rostral to the level of the preoptic area. It transmits olfactory information from the anterior olfactory nucleus on one side of the brain to the olfactory bulb and anterior olfactory nucleus of the contralateral side. The septal area (E), seen at this level of the forebrain as a thin structure separated by the lateral ventricles on both sides, receives major inputs from the hippocampal formation and is a principal component of the limbic system. The caudate nucleus (A), and the putamen, constitute the principal structures for receipt of afferent fibers. Primary sources of such input include the cerebral cortex and centromedian (CM) nucleus of the thalamus.

Motor Systems

DIRECTIONS: Each question below contains five suggested responses. Select the **one best** response to each question.

439. A patient presents with the following: she delays in initiating movement, displays an uneven trajectory in moving her hand from above her head to touch her nose, and is uneven in her attempts to demonstrate rapid alternation of pronating and supernating movements of the hand and forearm. She probably has a lesion in the:

(A) hemispheres of the posterior cerebellar lobe

(B) flocculonodular lobe of the cerebellum

(C) vermal region of the anterior cerebellar lobe

(D) fastigial nucleus

(E) ventral spinocerebellar tract

440. A tumor which invades the left motor cortex will damage cortical neurons that project directly (monosynaptically) to all of the following structures EXCEPT:

(A) ventral horn cells of the right side of the spinal cord

(B) cells in the deep pontine nuclei of the left side

(C) red nucleus cells of the left side

(D) right cerebellum

(E) cells of the ventrolateral (VL) nucleus of the left thalamus

441. Normal motor function of the cerebral cortex requires inputs from all of the following EXCEPT:

(A) cerebellum

(B) basal ganglia

(C) posterior parietal lobule

(D) mediodorsal nucleus

(E) ventral posterolateral nucleus (VPL)

442. In studying the functional relationships between motor cortex and spinal cord, which of the following effects of cortical stimulation on synaptic potentials would an investigator be likely to observe:

(A) the largest potentials would be seen in spinal motor neurons innervating proximal muscles

(B) the largest potentials would be seen in spinal motor neurons innervating distal muscles

(C) the potentials seen in spinal motor neurons innervating both proximal and distal muscles would be approximately equivalent

(D) the largest potentials would be seen in spinal sensory neurons carrying information from spindle afferents to the cerebellum

(E) the largest potentials would be seen in spinal sensory neurons carrying information from proprioceptors to the thalamus

443. Which of the following statements correctly characterizes properties of neurons in the motor cortex:

(A) In the resting state, the membranes of motor cortex neurons are more permeable to sodium than to potassium ions.

(B) Motor cortex neurons receive information from the muscle to which they project or from a region of skin related to the function of that muscle.

(C) Motor cortex neurons have reciprocal connections with the red nucleus.

(D) Motor cortex neurons that excite alpha motor neurons generally have little effect upon gamma motor neurons that project to the same muscle group.

(E) Motor neurons of the cerebral cortex have reciprocal, monosynaptic connections with neurons in the cerebellar cortex.

444. Spasticity may result from a lesion of:

(A) ventral horn cells

(B) corpus callosum

(C) postcentral gyrus

(D) internal capsule

(E) substantia nigra

445. Paralysis of the right side of the lower face, right spastic paralysis of the limbs, deviation of the tongue to the right with no atrophy, and no loss of taste from any region of tongue will likely result from a lesion of the

(A) internal capsule of the right side

(B) internal capsule of the left side

(C) right pontine tegmentum

(D) base of the medulla on right side

(E) base of the medulla on left side

446. All of the following statements concerning neurons of the motor cortex are correct EXCEPT:

(A) Neurons in the primary motor cortex encode the extent of limb movement rather than the degree of force of movement.

(B) The direction of movement is most likely encoded by the excitation patterns of populations of neurons in the motor cortex.

(C) Cortical neurons that are responsible for producing movement receive sensory feedback from the limb undergoing that movement.

(D) Neurons in the motor cortex make direct (monosynaptic) excitatory connections with flexor motor neurons of the spinal cord.

(E) A cluster of cortical neurons may influence more than one muscle group.

447. An impairment in the ability to perform certain types of learned, complex movements (referred to as apraxia) usually results from a lesion of the:

(A) precentral gyrus

(B) postcentral gyrus

(C) premotor cortex

(D) prefrontal cortex

(E) cingulate gyrus

448. The overwhelming majority of fibers supplying the basal ganglia terminate in the:

(A) paleostriatum

(B) neostriatum

(C) subthalamic nucleus

(D) substantia nigra

(E) claustrum

449. Neurons in the neostriatum are:

(A) inhibited by gamma aminobutyric acid (GABA) which is released at corticostriate terminals

(B) excited by glutamate which is released at corticostriate terminals

(C) inhibited by substance P which is released at corticostriate terminals

(D) excited by acetylcholine which is released from hypothalamic-caudate terminals

(E) inhibited by gamma aminobutyric acid (GABA) which is released at nigrostriatal terminals

450. The primary transmitter released from terminals of both neostriatal and paleostriatal neurons is:

(A) glycine

(B) enkephalin

(C) dopamine

(D) gamma aminobutyric acid (GABA)

(E) glutamate

451. All of the following statements concerning the substantia nigra are correct EXCEPT:

(A) dopamine from the pars compacta is released from nigrostriatal terminals

(B) gamma aminobutyric acid (GABAergic) fibers from the pars reticulata terminate in the ventral anterior (VA) and ventrolateral (VL) nuclei of thalamus

(C) fibers from the striatum project to the pars reticulata of the substantia nigra and utilize gamma aminobutyric acid (GABA) as their transmitter

(D) loss of dopaminergic cells in the substantia nigra may lead to Parkinson's disease

(E) the substantia nigra contains large numbers of cholinergic neurons

452. Since motor dysfunctions associated with disturbances of basal ganglia are expressed on the contralateral side of the body, one concludes:

(A) the basal ganglia project fibers to the spinal cord that are crossed

(B) the basal ganglia project fibers to motor nuclei of the brainstem whose axons then project to the contralateral spinal cord

(C) the basal ganglia project fibers to structures that ultimately influence motor regions of the ipsilateral cerebral cortex

(D) the basal ganglia project axons to the cerebellum whose outputs are known to modulate the contralateral side of the body

(E) the basal ganglia project fibers directly to the contralateral motor cortex

453. In Huntington's disease, there is a loss of:

(A) dopamine in the neostriatum

(B) substance P in the substantia nigra

(C) acetylcholine and gamma aminobutyric acid in intrastriatal and cortical neurons

(D) serotonin in the neostriatum

(E) most of the pallidal neurons

454. Damage to the subthalamic nucleus will result in:

(A) torsion dystonia

(B) tremor at rest

(C) hemiballism

(D) spastic paralysis

(E) tardive dyskinesia

455. Drugs that have had some positive results in ameliorating choreiform movements are:

(A) acetylcholine blockers because there is an excess of this transmitter in the caudate nucleus

(B) dopamine blockers because there is too low a ratio of acetylcholine to dopamine in the neostriatum

(C) serotonin blockers because there is too low a ratio of serotonin to acetylcholine and dopamine in the neostriatum

(D) substance P antagonists because the ratio of substance P to acetylcholine is too high in the neostriatum

(E) norepinephrine antagonists because the ratio of norepinephrine to acetylcholine is too high in the subthalamic nucleus

456. Tardive dyskinesia is most likely the result of:

(A) a change in serotonin receptors causing a hypersensitivity to serotonin

(B) a change in acetylcholine receptors causing a hypersensitivity to acetylcholine

(C) a change in enkephalin receptors causing a hypersensitivity to enkephalin

(D) a change in dopamine receptors causing a hypersensitivity to dopamine

(E) a change in gamma amino butyric acid (GABA) receptors causing a hypersensitivity to GABA

457. The neurotoxin MPTP (1-methyl-4-phenyl-1, 2, 3, 6-tetahydropyridine) has recently been applied experimentally with considerable success as a model for:

(A) Huntington's disease

(B) hemiballism

(C) Parkinson's disease

(D) tardive dyskinesia

(E) dystonia

458. The major afferent input to the flocculonodular lobe is from the:

(A) nucleus dorsalis of Clarke of the spinal cord

(B) red nucleus

(C) vestibular nuclei

(D) cerebral cortex

(E) midbrain reticular formation

459. The dorsal spinocerebellar tract, the ventral spinocerebellar tract, and the cuneocerebellar tract, in a general sense, show convergence in their projections to the cerebellum. The principal region within the cerebellum where these fibers converge is the:

(A) anterior lobe

(B) posterior lobe

(C) flocculonodular lobe

(D) fastigial nucleus

(E) dentate nucleus

460. Information arising from the cerebral cortex is known to reach the cerebellum. The fibers carrying it are:

(A) somatotopically distributed only to the anterior lobe

(B) somatotopically distributed only to the vermal region of the anterior and posterior lobes

(C) somatotopically distributed to the cerebellar hemispheres

(D) not somatotopically organized but do project to the hemispheres of the anterior and posterior lobes

(E) distributed mainly to the interposed and dentate nuclei

461. A cerebellar glomerulus includes:

(A) mossy fiber terminals, Golgi axons, and axon terminals of granule cells

(B) climbing fiber terminals, Golgi axons, and granule cell dendrites

(C) mossy fiber terminals, Purkinje cell axons, and granule cell dendrites

(D) mossy fiber terminals, Golgi and granule cell dendrites, and Golgi cell axon terminals

(E) climbing fiber terminals, Golgi cell dendrites, Purkinje cell dendrites, and axon terminals of parallel fibers

Questions 462-464. The cerebellum contains a number of important feedback relationships with different regions of the central nervous system. In each of the circuits listed below, one or more of the structures has been omitted. Indicate the structure(s) that must be added to complete that circuit.

462. Frontal lobe ——> deep pontine nuclei ——>cerebellar cortex ——> ___?___ ——> ___?___ ——>motor cortex (frontal lobe).

(A) fastigial nucleus ——>red nucleus

(B) interposed nuclei ——>red nucleus

(C) dentate nucleus ——>ventrolateral (VL) nucleus of the thalamus

(D) dentate nucleus ——>ventral anterior (VA) nucleus of the thalamus

(E) Purkinje cell axons ——>reticular formation of pons

463. Red nucleus ——> inferior olivary nucleus ——>cerebellar cortex of anterior and posterior lobes ——> ___?___ ——>red nucleus.

(A) fastigial nucleus

(B) interposed nuclei

(C) dentate nucleus

(D) Purkinje cells of cerebellar hemispheres

(E) vestibular nuclei

464. Spinal cord (via dorsal and ventral spinocerebellar tracts) ——> anterior lobe of cerebellum ——> ___?___ ——> reticular formation and vestibular nuclei ——> spinal cord.

(A) fastigial nucleus

(B) globose nucleus

(C) emboliform nucleus

(D) dentate nucleus

(E) red nucleus

465. All of the following concerning cerebellar Purkinje cells are true EXCEPT:

(A) they receive excitatory inputs from parallel fibers by way of axodendritic synapses

(B) they receive inhibitory inputs from basket cells by way of axosomatic synapses

(C) they receive excitatory inputs from climbing fibers which make axodendritic contacts along the dendritic tree of the Purkinje cell

(D) in the lateral third of the hemisphere they supply the fastigial nucleus

(E) the transmitter released from their axon terminals is gamma aminobutyric acid (GABA)

466. Based upon your knowledge of the anatomical and neurophysiological relationships of the anterior lobe of the cerebellum, you would predict that electrical stimulation of the medial vermal aspect of the cerebellar cortex of the anterior lobe will:

(A) produce rigidity

(B) produce spasticity

(C) cause tonic seizures to occur

(D) inhibit extensor muscle tone

(E) have little effect upon muscle tone

467. A patient presents with a wide-based, ataxic gait during his attempts at walking. He also is unsteady and sways when standing and displays a tendency to fall backward or to either side in a drunken manner. A lesion is most likely located in the:

(A) hemispheres of the posterior cerebellar lobe

(B) anterior limb of the internal capsule

(C) dentate nucleus

(D) anterior lobe of the cerebellum

(E) flocculonodular lobe of the cerebellum

Motor Systems

Answers

439. The answer is A. (Carpenter and Sutin, 3rd Ed., pp. 489-490) The classical appearance of an individual with a lesion of the cerebellar hemispheres is one in which voluntary and skilled movements are affected. They are uncoordinated and there are errors in the range, force, and direction of movement. The relationships between the cerebellum and the motor regions of the cerebral cortex have been disrupted. Lesions of other regions such as the flocculonodular lobe, vermal region of the anterior cerebellar cortex, or fastigial nucleus produce different symptoms (disturbances of balance, muscle tone, or nystagmus). Although "pure" lesions limited to the ventral spinocerebellar tract have not been reported, it is likely that such a lesion could not account for the symptoms indicated in this question. Information carried by this tract concerns activity of Golgi tendon organs of muscles of the lower limbs.

440. The answer is D. (Carpenter and Sutin, 8th Ed., pp. 433-434, 684-689, 694-697) It is extremely important to note that fibers from the motor cortex are directed not only to the spinal cord but also to a number of other target structures associated with the regulation of motor functions. These include the red nucleus (as part of a corticorubral - rubrospinal system), ventrolateral (VL) nucleus of the thalamus (as part of a feedback mechanism regulating cortical afferents from the basal ganglia and cerebellum), and deep pontine nuclei (as part of a cortico-pontine-cerebellar pathway). Projections to brainstem nuclei mentioned in this question are ipsilateral, while the projection to the spinal cord is principally contralateral. The pathway from the cerebral cortex to the cerebellum is not a direct one. It involves an initial synapse in the deep pontine nuclei whose axons then project to the contralateral cerebellar cortex.

441. The answer is D. (Kandel, 3rd Ed., pp. 610-623) In order for functions of the corticospinal tract to be properly executed, the cell bodies of these descending fiber groups require inputs from all of the regions listed in this question. Priming and feedback functions are provided by the basal ganglia and cerebellum. Important sensory feedback concerning position sense (which is essential for appropriate motor adjustments) is generated from the dorsal column-medial lemniscal system via ventral posterolateral nucleus of the thalamus (VPL). Finally, the programming or sequencing of the response mechanism is regulated by inputs into the premotor region from the posterior parietal lobe and ventral anterior thalamic nucleus (VA). Without inputs from the posterior parietal lobe, the performance of complex motor tasks would not be possible. The mediodorsal thalamic nucleus integrates information associated with limbic system structures, including the prefrontal cortex and is not directly associated with the regulation of motor functions.

442. The answer is B. (Kandel, 3rd Ed., pp. 612-613; Carpenter and Sutin, 8th Ed., pp. 252-253, 282-289) The largest synaptic potentials produced by cortical stimulation would most likely be seen in spinal motor neurons that innervate distal muscles. One of the primary functions of the corticospinal tract is to control the distal muscles of the hand and fingers. Penfield and others constructed a homuncular map from stimulation studies of the cortex. Such studies reveal that the region of cortex associated with the hand and fingers is considerably larger than those regions associated with the proximal musculature. Accordingly, stimulation of the hand region of cortex would activate more fibers than other cortical regions. It is likely that more ventral horn neurons (located in a lateral position) innervate distal musculature than neurons (located in a medial position) innervate proximal musculature. Since the size of the synaptic potential is a function of both the number of fibers that provide a converging input into a given region and the numbers of cells that discharge in response to that converging input, it is reasonable to conclude that the largest potentials would be observed following stimulation of the cortical regions associated with the distal musculature. Since neurons situated in the motor cortex project their axons to motor horn cells and (interneurons) but not to sensory neurons of the dorsal horn (although the component of the corticospinal tract arising from the parietal lobe does project to the dorsal horn), stimulation of the motor cortex could only produce weak potentials (at best) among sensory neurons in the dorsal horn.

443. The answer is B. (Kandel, pp. 105-111, 613-623) Motor cortex neurons receive information from the muscle to which they project or from a region of skin related to the function of that muscle. The anatomical pathway includes dorsal column-medial lemniscal fibers that terminate in the ventral posterolateral (VPL) nucleus of the thalamus. Fibers from VPL then project to the postcentral gyrus. Fibers from a given region of the primary sensory cortex project to the region of primary motor cortex whose projection target in the spinal cord involves the same muscle group (or body part) from which the sensory stimulus originated. All other choices are incorrect. The properties of membrane potentials of neurons in the motor cortex follow the same principles as those found elsewhere in the nervous system; namely, that, in the resting state, the cell membrane is more permeable to potassium than to sodium. The red nucleus does not have an ascending projection (and, therefore, cannot be reciprocally connected with the motor cortex). Its fibers project, instead, to the spinal cord and lower brainstem. In general, corticospinal fibers that activate alpha motor neurons which innervate a given muscle group will also synapse with gamma motor neurons associated with that same muscle group. Coactivation of both alpha and gamma motor neurons is an important principle because it enables muscle spindles to react to changes in the length of the muscle even during the process of movement of the limb associated with that muscle. The projection to the cerebellum from the motor cortex is disynaptic. Projections from the cerebellum to the motor cortex synapse in the dentate nucleus and the ventrolateral nucleus of the thalamus.

444. The answer is D. (Carpenter and Sutin, 8th Ed., pp. 288, 688) An upper motor neuron paralysis occurs following a lesion of the internal capsule. Such a lesion disrupts not only fibers destined for the spinal cord but others that project to parts of the reticular formation and activate inhibitory reticulospinal mechanisms. Loss of such inhibitory input to spinal cord motor neurons then leads to increased levels of excitation of these neurons. The behavioral manifestation of this process is spasticity. Lesions of ventral horn cells produce a flaccid paralysis. Lesions of the postcentral gyrus primarily produce sensory loss, not spasticity. Since the corpus callosum is concerned with interhemispheric transfer of information, a lesion of this bundle will not produce spasticity. A lesion of the substantia nigra will result in Parkinson's disease, which is associated with tremors at rest and rigidity, but not spasticity.

445. The answer is B. (Carpenter and Sutin, 8th Ed., pp. 274, 352-354, 536-538, 685-696) This constellation of deficits, including paralysis of the lower right face, paralysis of right lower limbs, and right deviation of the tongue, requires a lesion located in the left internal capsule. Since the motor fibers from the cortex that supply all three of these regions (i.e., limbs, lower face, and tongue) are all crossed, a lesion of the internal capsule will produce each of these deficits. Also, recall that the tongue will deviate to the side of the lesion when the lesion affects the lower motor neuron (i.e., cranial nerve XII) directly. When it affects the upper motor neuron (i.e., fibers in the internal capsule), inputs into the contralateral nucleus of cranial nerve XII are affected. Thus, the tongue in this instance will deviate to the side opposite the lesion. A lesion of the pontine tegmentum will not affect descending corticospinal or cortico-medullary fibers since these fibers are contained in the basilar part of the pons. A lesion of the medulla would be too caudal to affect cortical fibers that terminate on cells of the facial nucleus whose axons innervate muscles of the lower face.

446. The answer is A. (Kandel, 3rd Ed., pp. 610-619) Experiments conducted by Evarts have shown that neurons in the primary motor cortex can respond to proprioceptive stimuli. For example, these neurons encode the amount of force of the movement rather than the extent of the movement. This was demonstrated when motor cortex neurons discharged much more rapidly when the wrist had to be flexed under a load than when the load was not present although the extent of movement in both cases was the same. It has been demonstrated that the direction of movement is not encoded by a single neuron, Each neuron responds to movement regardless of direction (although it may be most sensitive to movement in one particular direction). Thus, the direction of movement is encoded by the sum total of the activity of many neurons. Motor neurons receive sensory feedback signals from regions of the body with which those neurons are functionally and anatomically associated. Moreover, descending motor neurons from the cortex can directly excite flexor motor neurons of the spinal cord (without involving interneurons). In addition, single cortical neurons may affect several muscle groups. Conversely, a single muscle group may be represented by several clusters of cortical neurons.

447. The answer is C. (Kandel, 3rd Ed., pp. 619-621) The premotor areas play an important role in the programming or sequencing of responses that comprise complex learned movements. They receive significant inputs for this process from the posterior parietal lobule and in turn signal appropriate neurons in the brainstem and spinal cord (both flexors and extensors). Lesions of the postcentral gyrus produce a somatosensory loss. Lesions of the precentral gyrus produce paralysis. Neither lesions of the prefrontal cortex nor the cingulate gyrus have been reported to produce apraxia.

448. The answer is B. (Kandel, 3rd Ed., pp. 648-650) The neostriatum (i.e., caudate nucleus and putamen) constitutes the principal, if not exclusive, receiving area for afferent fibers to the basal ganglia. The subthalamic nucleus and the substantia nigra share reciprocal connections with the paleostriatum (i.e., globus pallidus) and the neostriatum, respectively. However, these areas receive few, if any, fibers from the cerebral cortex or the centromedian nucleus of the thalamus, which are the major afferent sources to the basal ganglia. Functions of the claustrum are not well understood, but it is believed to be more closely associated with the neocortex than with the basal ganglia.

449. The answer is B. (Kandel, 3rd Ed., pp. 652-654) The cerebral cortex is a principal source of afferent fibers to the neostriatum and it utilizes glutamate as its transmitter, which is excitatory to caudate neurons. Thus, neither gamma aminobutyric acid (GABA) nor substance P are transmitters from the cortex to the neostriatum; neither is GABA a transmitter released from the nigrostriatal terminals. Projections from the hypothalamus to the caudate nucleus have never been demonstrated and, presumably, do not exist.

450. The answer is D. (Kandel, 3rd Ed., pp. 652-654) The major transmitter released at terminals of neostriatal and paleostriatal fibers is gamma aminobutyric acid (GABA) . Thus, the output of the basal ganglia is mainly inhibitory. This suggests that thalamic influences upon the cortex are generated through the process of disinhibition whereby neurons of the basal ganglia are inhibited. The presence of glycine in striatal neurons has yet to be demonstrated. Enkephalins are released from terminals of neostriatal-pallidal fibers but not from other efferent neurons of the striatum. Dopamine is released from brainstem and some adjoining hypothalamic neurons but certainly not from striatal neurons. The neostriatum receives cortical inputs which utilize glutamate, but the release of GABA from terminals of striatal efferent fibers has not been demonstrated.

451. The answer is E. (Kandel, 3rd Ed., pp. 652-655; Carpenter and Sutin, 8th Ed., pp. 448-453, 590-591) Dopaminergic fibers from the pars compacta of the nigra supply the neostriatum, When these fibers are damaged or the cells of origin destroyed, the result is Parkinson's disease. Fibers from the neo- and paleostriatum project GABAergic fibers (release gamma aminobutyric acid) to the pars reticulata of the substantia nigra. The neurons of the pars reticulata are also GABAergic and their projections are to the ventrolateral (VL) and ventral anterior (VA) nuclei of the thalamus. There is no evidence to support the notion that large numbers of cholinergic neurons are present in any part of the substantia nigra.

452. The answer is C. (Kandel, 3rd Ed., pp. 652-655) The basic principle governing how the basal ganglia control motor activity is that they do so by modulating neurons of the motor cortex and premotor areas (of the ipsilateral side) via synaptic connections in the ventrolateral (VL) and ventral anterior (VA) nuclei of the thalamus. One can see from the circuits:

globus pallidus   —>   ventrolateral nucleus   —>   area 4 of cortex
(medial segment)   (VL)

globus pallidus   —>   ventral anterior nucleus   —>   area 6 of cortex
(medial segment)   (VA)

that damage to the basal ganglia on one side of the brain will affect cortical neurons on the same side. This will result in dyskinesia expressed on the contralateral side of the body because the corticospinal tract is crossed. The other possibilities listed in the question are not viable. Projections of the basal ganglia to brainstem nuclei are minimal. The basal ganglia do not project fibers down to the spinal cord nor do they project to the cerebellum.

453. The answer is C. (Kandel, 3rd Ed., pp. 654-657; Carpenter and Sutin, 8th Ed., p. 608) In Huntington's disease, the essential neurochemical change is in the basal ganglia where there is a significant reduction in the two transmitters, acetylcholine and gamma aminobutyric acid (GABA). In particular, there are reduced levels of choline acetyltransferase, glutamic acid decarboxylase, and GABA.

454. The answer is C. (Kandel, 3rd Ed., pp. 654-656; Carpenter and Sutin, 8th Ed., pp. 608-609) A lesion of the subthalamic nucleus results in hemiballism, a form of dyskinesia in which the patient displays severe involuntary movements. It is believed to occur as a result of an imbalance in the output signals of the basal ganglia. There is a change in the relationship between efferent pathways associated with the two pallidal segments (i.e., a direct pathway from the medial pallidal segment to the ventrolateral (VL) and ventroanterior (VA) nuclei of the thalamus versus an indirect pathway, involving connections between the lateral pallidal segment, subthalamic nucleus, and substantia nigra). Thus, in hemiballism, the indirect pathway is disrupted, resulting in a change in the output signals of the pallidum to the thalamus.

455. The answer is B. (Carpenter and Sutin, 8th Ed., p. 608; Kandel, 3rd Ed., p. 654) Choreiform movements have generally been associated with damage to the neostriatum (the cortex and the globus pallidus have occasionally been implicated). Normally, there is a balance in what seems to be opposing effects of acetylcholine, dopamine, and gamma amino butyric acid (GABA) in the neostriatum. In this disorder, the levels of acetylcholine and GABA are significantly reduced. This creates an imbalance in which dopamine levels now become (relatively) too high. Accordingly, effective pharmacological treatment involves the use of dopamine receptor blockers.

456. The answer is D. (Kandel, 3rd Ed., pp. 654-657) Tardive dyskinesia, a disorder involving involuntary movements of the mouth, face, and tongue, is caused by long-term treatment with antipsychotic drugs that block or decrease dopaminergic synaptic transmission. Such treatment eventually produces a hypersensitivity in dopamine receptors to dopamine. An imbalance is created between dopamine, gamma amino butyric acid (GABA), and cholinergic systems within the striatum which is believed to be responsible for the disorder.

457. The answer is C. (Kandel, 3rd Ed., pp. 655-656) MPTP (1-methyl-4-phenyl-1,2,3,6-tetahydropyridine) was discovered by accident when drug abusers, who were using a synthetic heroin derivative, developed signs of Parkinson's disease. It was discovered that their drug included the contaminant MPTP. As a consequence, MPTP has been applied systemically in a number of experimental animals, resulting in significant decreases in dopamine content of the brain due to the loss of dopaminergic neurons in the substantia nigra. These animals also developed symptoms similar to those seen in Parkinson's patients. For these reasons, this drug is currently being utilized for research purposes in order to develop a better understanding of this disease and to establish possible drug therapies for its treatment and eventual cure.

458. The answer is C. (Kandel, 3rd Ed., pp. 634-635) The principal source of afferent fibers to the flocculonodular lobe is the vestibular complex, in particular, the inferior and medial vestibular nuclei. For this reason, this lobe of the cerebellum is sometimes referred to as the "vestibulocerebellum." The red nucleus and cerebral cortex project topographically (via relays in the inferior olivary nucleus and deep pontine nuclei, respectively) to the anterior and posterior lobes. Pathways arising from the spinal cord such as the spinocerebellar tract project to the anterior lobe. Other fibers arising from the spinal cord enter the cerebellum through a relay in the inferior olivary nucleus. Such fibers terminate in both anterior and posterior lobes.

459. The answer is A. (Carpenter and Sutin, 8th Ed., pp. 475-476) One of the most important features of the anterior lobe of the cerebellum is that it receives major inputs from structures that mediate information concerning muscle spindle and Golgi tendon organ activity (sometimes referred to as "unconscious proprioception"). The pathways that mediate unconscious proprioception include the dorsal and ventral spinocerebellar tracts and the cuneocerebellar tract. Accordingly, the cerebellar anterior lobe is sometimes referred to as the "spinocerebellum." The fastigial and dentate nuclei receive their principal inputs from the cerebellar cortex and their axons project out of the cerebellum. The posterior lobe receives few, if any, inputs from pathways that mediate unconscious proprioception information.

460. The answer is C. (Carpenter and Sutin, 8th Ed., pp. 476-477; Kandel, 3rd Ed., p. 635) A unique feature of the connections between cerebral cortex and the cerebellum is the somatotopically organized projection from the cerebral cortex largely to the cerebellar hemispheres (some fibers terminate in the vermis). The somatotopic maps are arranged in both anterior and posterior lobes in a manner that has the distal musculature functionally represented in the lateral aspect of the hemispheres while the proximal musculature is represented toward or in the vermal region. Because of this somatotopic arrangement, the lateral hemispheres are concerned with functions associated with detailed movements of the limbs, while more medial regions are concerned with regulation of the proximal musculature (e.g., postural mechanisms).

461. The answer is D. (Kandel, 3rd Ed., p. 630; Carpenter and Sutin, 8th Ed., p. 463) The cerebellar glomerulus consists of mossy fiber terminals, dendrites, axon terminals of Golgi cells, and granule cell dendrites. The flow of information in the glomerulus is as follows:

(1) information reaches the cerebellar cortex through mossy fibers.

(2) axon terminals of mossy fibers terminate upon dendrites of either granule or Golgi cells.

(3) collaterals of parallel fibers (axons of granule cells) may contact dendrites of Golgi cells whose axons then "feed back" onto the granule cells.

(4) mossy fiber terminals synapse with Golgi cell dendrites, whose axons then make synaptic contact with the granule cell ("feed forward" mechanism).

The axons of granule cells run parallel to the cortex and perpendicular to the orientation of the Purkinje cell dendrites with which they synapse. The circuitry for "feedback" and "feed forward" mechanisms are indicated below:

"feedback" mechanism:

mossy fiber axon terminal —> granule cell dendrites —> granule cell axon —> Golgi cell —> (inhibits) granule cell.

"feed forward" mechanism:

mossy fiber axon terminal —> Golgi cell dendrites —> Golgi cell axon —> (inhibits) granule cell.

462-464. The answers are: 462-C, 463-B, 464-A. (Kandel, 3rd Ed., pp. 632-636) For each of these questions, the central point relates to the projection targets of the relevant deep cerebellar nuclei and their relationship to their afferent sources. In Question 462, note that the inputs from the frontal lobe eventually reach the cerebellar cortex (which involves the cerebellar hemispheres of the anterior and posterior lobes to a large extent). Because many of these cerebellar afferents terminate in the lateral aspect of the hemisphere, the return (or feedback) pathway will initially involve Purkinje cell axons that synapse with cells in the dentate nucleus. Fibers of the dentate nucleus then supply the ventrolateral (VL) nucleus of the thalamus, which, in turn, supplies the primary motor cortex. Question 463 concerns the feedback pathways associated with the red nucleus. Inputs to the cerebellum from the red nucleus utilize the inferior olivary nucleus as a relay. These inputs supply the anterior and posterior cerebellar lobes in a topographic manner. Since many of these fibers are distributed to an intermediolateral position within the cerebellar cortex, Purkinje cells from this area supply the interposed (i.e., globose and emboliform) nuclei. The interposed nuclei, in turn, supply the red nucleus via the superior cerebellar peduncle. In Question 464, the issue concerns the relationship of the cerebellum to those spinal cord mechanisms relating to descending fibers of the vestibulospinal and reticulospinal systems. Recall that many of the spinocerebellar fibers are distributed to the medial vermal region of the anterior lobe. Thus, the return flow of information to the spinal cord with respect to the regulation of muscle tension will involve the vestibulospinal and reticulospinal systems. To achieve this objective, the Purkinje cells of the medial (vermal and paravermal) regions of cerebellar cortex project to the fastigial nucleus. The fastigial nucleus, in turn, projects to both the reticular formation and vestibular nuclei, which then complete the feedback circuit by sending their axons down to the spinal cord.

465. The answer is D. (Kandel, 3rd Ed., pp. 630-633; Carpenter and Sutin, 8th Ed., pp. 462-470) The projection pattern of Purkinje cell axons from the cerebellar cortex to the deep cerebellar nuclei is topographically organized. Purkinje cells situated along the medial aspect of the cortex, including the vermal region, project to the fastigial nucleus. Purkinje cells in an intermediolateral region of the cerebellar cortex project their axons to the interposed nuclei, and those located in the lateral aspect of the cerebellar cortex project to the dentate nucleus (not the fastigial nucleus). Other statements in this question are correct. Purkinje cells receive excitatory inputs from parallel and climbing fibers and inhibitory inputs from basket cells. They are inhibitory neurons and utilize gamma aminobutyric acid (GABA) as a neurotransmitter.

466. The answer is D. (Carpenter and Sutin, 8th Ed., pp. 490-491) This experiment was actually carried out many years ago by Sherrington. He observed that stimulation of the medial vermal region of the cerebellar cortex resulted in inhibition of extensor muscle tone. It is most likely that stimulation directly activated local populations of Purkinje cells which then inhibited the fastigial nucleus. Since the fastigial nucleus (as well as the other deep cerebellar nuclei) has excitatory effects upon its target neurons, inhibition of the fastigial nucleus following local stimulation of the cerebellar cortex would result in decreased activation of the vestibulospinal system. Thus, such a mechanism could account for the inhibition of muscle tone seen after stimulation of the anterior vermal region of cortex.

467. The answer is E. (Carpenter and Sutin, 8th Ed., p. 490) Since the flocculonodular lobe receives and integrates inputs from the vestibular system, it is understandable why lesions which disrupt this integrating mechanism for vestibular inputs would result in difficulties in maintaining balance. Indeed, this is a classical feature of lesions of the flocculonodular lobe but is not associated with lesions in the hemispheres of the posterior lobe, anterior limb of the internal capsule, or the dentate nucleus, which are functionally linked to the frontal lobe. Lesions of the anterior lobe also do not affect mechanisms controlling balance.

Higher Functions

Questions 468-478

(A) ventral anterior thalamic nucleus

(B) ventrolateral thalamic nucleus

(C) centromedian thalamic nucleus

(D) pulvinar

(E) mediodorsal thalamic nucleus

(F) lateral geniculate thalamic nucleus

(G) medial geniculate thalamic nucleus

(H) anterior nucleus of the thalamus

(I) ventral posteromedial thalamic nucleus

(J) ventral posterolateral thalamic nucleus

(K) habenula complex

468. stimulation frequency of 6-12 Hz produces a cortical recruiting response

469. maintains reciprocal connections with the prefrontal cortex

470. utilizes the stria medullaris as a primary afferent pathway

471. receives inputs from the mammillary bodies and fornix

472. projects its fibers to the ventrolateral aspect of the postcentral gyrus

473. projects axons to the dorsomedial aspect of the postcentral gyrus

474. projects extensively to the inferior parietal lobule and receives tertiary auditory and visual inputs

475. projects axons to area 17 of the cerebral cortex

476. projects axons to areas 41 and 42 of the cerebral cortex

477. projects in a diffuse manner to the frontal cortex and receives inputs from the substantia nigra and globus pallidus

478. projects to the neostriatum

Questions 479-483

    (A) alpha waves

    (B) beta waves

    (C) delta waves

    (D) response characterized by very high frequency and amplitude

    (E) low frequency (2-4/s.), rectangular wave

479. EEG during stage 4 of slow wave sleep

480. EEG when alert

481. EEG during grand mal epilepsy

482. EEG during a focal seizure

483. EEG during states of quiet wakefulness

DIRECTIONS: Each question below contains five suggested responses. Select the **one best** response to each question.

484. Vasopressin is released from the posterior pituitary. However, it is synthesized in the:

(A) mammillary bodies

(B) lateral hypothalamus

(C) supraoptic hypothalamic nucleus

(D) ventromedial hypothalamic nucleus

(E) posterior hypothalamus

485. All of the following statements concerning the medial forebrain bundle are correct EXCEPT:

(A) cells located in the septal area contribute to the medial forebrain bundle

(B) cells located in parts of the amygdala contribute to the medial forebrain bundle

(C) hypothalamic cells contribute descending fibers in the medial forebrain bundle to the brainstem

(D) the medial forebrain bundle is located within the medial hypothalamus

(E) the medial forebrain bundle contains both ascending and descending fibers

486. The supraoptic nucleus is most closely associated with:

(A) feeding behavior

(B) temperature regulation

(C) sexual behavior

(D) short-term memory functions

(E) water balance

487. Afferent fibers which supply the hypothalamus arise from all of the following structures EXCEPT:

(A) ventral tegmental area

(B) substantia nigra

(C) medial septal nucleus

(D) basomedial amygdaloid nuclei

(E) raphe nuclei

488. All of the following are likely to occur as a result of a stressful event EXCEPT:

(A) glucocorticoids released from the adrenal gland

(B) increased response to a painful stimulus

(C) release of adrenocorticotrophic hormone (ACTH) from the pituitary

(D) sudden increase in blood pressure and heart rate

(E) sudden release of vasopressin

489. Electrical stimulation of the medial hypothalamus of the cat elicits all of the following events EXCEPT:

(A) increases in heart rate and blood pressure

(B) rage behavior

(C) feeding

(D) pupillary dilatation

(E) marked vocalization such as hissing

490. Which of the following statements concerning temperature regulation is correct:

(A) Stimulation of the posterior hypothalamus results in panting, dilation of blood vessels, and suppression of shivering.

(B) Neurons in the anterior hypothalamus respond to local warming of hypothalamic tissue but not to warming of the skin.

(C) Stimulation of the anterior hypothalamus may produce constriction of blood vessels and shivering.

(D) Neurons in the preoptic region and septal area act in concert to intensify increases in body temperature generated by pyrogens.

(E) Temperature regulation requires the integration of skeletomuscular, endocrine, and autonomic responses.

491. Lesions of the lateral hypothalamus will likely produce:

(A) feeding behaviors

(B) drinking behaviors

(C) sexual behaviors

(D) aphagia

(E) hypertension

492. A number of investigations have provided strong evidence that the suprachiasmatic nucleus plays an important role in:

(A) water intake

(B) food intake

(C) hypertension

(D) circadian rhythms

(E) short-term memory

493. The amygdala receives significant inputs from all of the following structures EXCEPT:

(A) prefrontal cortex

(B) cingulate gyrus

(C) hypothalamus

(D) locus ceruleus

(E) olfactory bulb

494. The Kluver-Bucy syndrome is typically associated with lesions of the:

(A) septal area

(B) amygdala

(C) cingulate gyrus

(D) medial hypothalamus

(E) lateral hypothalamus

495. The central nucleus of the amygdala:

(A) projects its axons to the medial hypothalamus via the stria terminalis

(B) is a major receiving area for information concerning tertiary auditory and visual signals

(C) has high concentrations of enkephalins, somatostatin, and dopamine

(D) is a primary location of norepinephrine-containing cell bodies in the forebrain

(E) projects axons which directly inhibit spinal motor neurons

496. A tumor that encroaches upon the hippocampal formation could likely result in each of the following dysfunctions EXCEPT:

(A) psychomotor epilepsy

(B) loss of emotional stability

(C) deviations from normal endocrine function

(D) loss of ability to regulate body temperature

(E) short-term memory loss

497. While the hippocampal formation has few if any direct (monosynaptic) connections with the lateral hypothalamus, it is known to modulate functions associated with the hypothalamus. The underlying anatomical substrate for such effects is mediated via a synaptic relay in the:

(A) cingulate gyrus

(B) habenular nucleus

(C) mediodorsal thalamic nucleus

(D) septal area

(E) bed nucleus of the stria terminalis

498. Which of the following comprises the Papez circuit:

(A) hippocampal formation —> mammillary bodies —> anterior thalamic nucleus —> prefrontal cortex —> hippocampal formation

(B) hippocampal formation —> septal area —> hypothalamus —> hippocampal formation

(C) hippocampal formation —> mammillary bodies —> anterior thalamic nucleus —> cingulate gyrus —> hippocampal formation

(D) amygdala —> hippocampal formation —> mammillary bodies —> amygdala

(E) prefrontal cortex —> hippocampal formation —> septal area —> medial hypothalamus —> prefrontal cortex

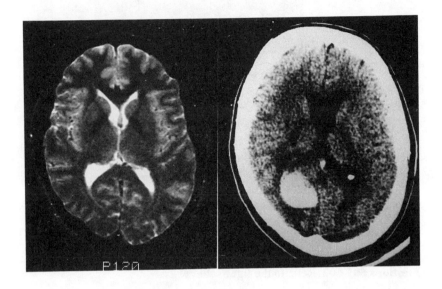

(Courtesy of Alan Zimmer, M.D.)

Questions 499-500 Refer to the figure above.

499. The T2-weighted MRI scan on the left side of the figure above is of a normal individual. In the CT scan on the right side, the patient had sustained a right cerebral hemorrhage, indicated by the large white area. It is likely that the cerebrovascular accident produced:

(A) right homonymous hemianopsia

(B) left homonymous hemianopsia

(C) loss of intellectual and emotional processes

(D) aphasia

(E) hemiparesis of the right side of the body

500. The blood vessel affected in the figure above is the:

(A) anterior cerebral artery

(B) middle cerebral artery

(C) posterior cerebral artery

(D) superior cerebellar artery

(E) striate arteries

R   L

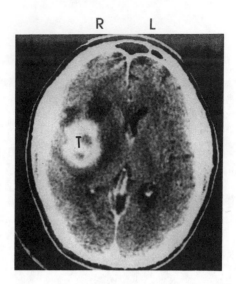

(Courtesy of Alan Zimmer, M.D.)

Questions 501-502 Refer to the figure above.

501. The CT scan above reveals that an individual has a glioma (T) on the right side of the brain. It is likely that the individual has sustained:

(A) an upper motor neuron paralysis of the left side

(B) dyskinesia

(C) intention tremor

(D) upper left quadrantanopia

(E) upper right quadrantanopia

502. The tumor in the scan above has most likely damaged the:

(A) lentiform nucleus only

(B) internal capsule only

(C) thalamus only

(D) lentiform nucleus and internal capsule

(E) lentiform nucleus, internal capsule, and thalamus

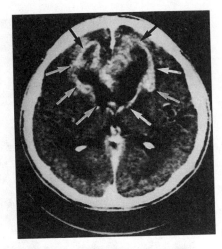

(Courtesy of Alan Zimmer, M.D.)

Questions 503-504 Refer to the figure above.

503. The contrast enhanced CT scan above reveals the presence of an extensive glioblastoma (arrows). The patient likely presents with all of the following symptoms EXCEPT:

(A) a loss of ability to solve complex problems (e.g. delayed alternation task)

(B) bilateral upper motor neuron paralysis

(C) marked changes in affect

(D) seizures

(E) perseveration on a card-sorting task

504. As a result of the tumor in the scan above, there will be significant loss of inputs from the tumor region to all the following structures EXCEPT:

(A) mediodorsal thalamic nucleus

(B) basilar portion of the pons

(C) amygdala

(D) neostriatum

(E) lateral geniculate thalamic nucleus

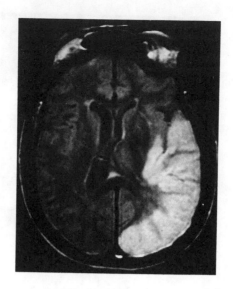

(Courtesy of Alan Zimmer, M.D.)

Questions 505-506 Refer to the figure above.

505. This patient whose CT scan is in the figure above sustained an occlusion of a major artery on the left side of the brain. The most prominent deficits will most likely include:

(A) a right homonymous hemianopsia only

(B) aphasia only

(C) a right homonymous hemianopsia coupled with aphasia

(D) marked intellectual deficits

(E) marked intellectual deficits coupled with hemiballism

506. The blood vessel occluded in the figure above is the:

(A) anterior cerebral artery

(B) middle cerebral artery

(C) posterior cerebral artery

(D) posterior choroidal artery

(E) superior cerebellar artery

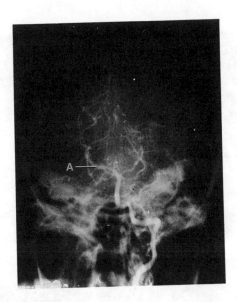

(Courtesy of Alan Zimmer, M.D.)

Questions 507-508   Refer to the figure above.

507. The vertebral angiogram in the figure above reveals the effects of a severe motorcycle accident upon a 21-year-old female. As a result of the accident, she most likely suffers from:

(A) an upper motor neuron paralysis of the right side of the body

(B) a right homonymous hemianopsia

(C) a left upper quadrantanopia

(D) aphasia

(E) dyskinesia

508. The artery occluded on the left side and shown at (A) in the figure above on the normal side is:

(A) vertebral

(B) basilar

(C) middle cerebral

(D) anterior cerebral

(E) posterior cerebral

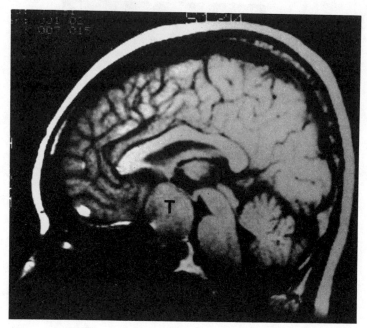

Question 509 Refer to the figure above.

509. The MRI in the figure above reveals a large chromophobe adenoma (T) of the pituitary that impinges on the adjoining brain tissue. This tumor caused a:

(A) binasal hemianopsia

(B) loss of the pupillary light reflex

(C) loss of the accommodation reflex

(D) bitemporal hemianopsia

(E) loss of conjugate gaze

Higher Functions

Answers

468-478. The answers are: 468-C, 469-E, 470-K, 471-H, 472-I, 473-J, 474-D, 475-F, 476-G, 477-A, 478-C. (Carpenter and Sutin, 8th Ed., pp. 508-509, 545-550) Stimulation of the centromedian nucleus (C) at 6-12 Hz will produce a recruiting response over widespread areas of the cortex. This response is characterized by a waxing and waning of the signal over an extended period of time. The centromedian nucleus is also a principal source of fibers from the thalamus to the neostriatum. The mediodorsal thalamic nucleus (E) is of considerable importance because of its relationships with the prefrontal cortex with which it maintains reciprocal connections. The habenula complex (K), located at the roof of the posterior aspect of the thalamus, receives afferent fibers which reach it by passing through the stria medullaris. The anterior nucleus (H) of the thalamus is part of the Papez circuit and thus receives inputs from both mammillary bodies and fornix (i.e., hippocampal formation). The ventral posteromedial nucleus (I) is part of the somatosensory pathway for the head region and thus receives somatosensory inputs from the main and spinal nuclei of the trigeminal complex. The ventral posterolateral nucleus (J) projects somatosensory information from the body region to the primary sensory cortex for the body region that is located on the dorsal aspect of the postcentral gyrus. The pulvinar nucleus (D) projects extensively to the inferior parietal lobule and receives inputs from portions of the occipital and temporal lobes associated with the integration of visual and auditory signals. The lateral geniculate nucleus (F) is a cortical relay nucleus for the visual system and therefore projects its axons to the primary visual cortex located in area 17. Similarly, the medial geniculate nucleus (G) projects its axons to the primary auditory receiving portions of cortex located in areas 41 and 42 of the superior temporal gyrus. The ventral anterior nucleus (A), linked with motor functions of the basal ganglia, receives significant inputs from the globus pallidus and substantia nigra, and projects its axons in a diffuse manner to wide areas of the frontal lobe, including (in particular) the premotor cortex (area 6).

479-483. The answers are: 479-C, 480-B, 481-D, 482-E, 483-A. (Guyton, 2nd Ed., pp. 268-270) The EEG response changes during different stages of sleep. In stage 4 of sleep, the EEG frequency becomes very slow with a frequency of approximately 3.5/s. or less. This pattern is called a delta wave. When an individual is alert, the EEG contains beta waves (B) which are characterized by low voltage, high frequency (>14 Hz). The EEG typical of grand mal epilepsy has a very high frequency and very high amplitude (D). This is contrasted with the EEG during focal or psychomotor epilepsy in which the waves are low frequency (2-4/s.) and rectangular in shape (E). Occasionally, a higher frequency wave is superimposed over the slow waves. During states of quiet wakefulness or drowsiness, the EEG pattern becomes slower (8-13 Hz; average amplitude of 50 V) than what is seen during an alert state. This pattern is called an alpha wave (A).

484. The answer is C. (Kandel, 3rd Ed., p. 744) Certain magnocellular neurons of the hypothalamus synthesize the hormones vasopressin and oxytocin. These include the paraventricular and supraoptic nuclei. The cell bodies of the magnocellular neurons producing vasopressin are found mostly within the supraoptic nucleus. Vasopressin is important because it makes the membranes of the convoluted tubules and collecting ducts of the kidneys more permeable to water. This results in water conservation.

485. The answer is D. (Carpenter and Sutin, 8th Ed., pp. 560, 584) The significant feature of the medial forebrain bundle is that it not only conveys descending fibers from limbic and lateral hypothalamic nuclei (through the lateral hypothalamus) to the brainstem tegmentum, but it also conveys information that passes in a rostral direction from the lateral hypothalamus to several limbic nuclei. These rostrally directed fibers serve as possible feedback mechanisms which could assist limbic structures in their modulation of hypothalamic processes. In addition, other ascending fibers, which arise from brainstem nuclei, such as the midbrain periaqueductal gray, midbrain tegmentum, and monoaminergic nuclei, utilize the medial forebrain bundle to supply wide regions of the forebrain, including the cerebral cortex.

486. The answer is E. (Kandel, 3rd Ed., p. 744) The supraoptic nucleus, like the paraventricular nucleus, contains magnocellular neurons which synthesize vasopressin and oxytocin and transport these hormones down their axons to the posterior pituitary. For this reason, the supraoptic nucleus plays a significant role in the regulation of water balance. There is no evidence to support the notion that the supraoptic nucleus has a role in feeding behavior, temperature regulation, sexual behavior, or short-term memory functions.

487. The answer is B. (Carpenter and Sutin, 8th Ed., pp. 560-564) Ventral tegmental neurons project their axons to the mammillary bodies, and, in addition, may contribute dopaminergic fibers to wide areas of the hypothalamus as they do to other parts of the forebrain. The substantia nigra has no known projection to the hypothalamus. There are two principal projections of the substantia nigra — dopaminergic fibers to the neostriatum and GABAergic fibers to the ventral anterior (VA) and ventrolateral (VL) thalamic nuclei. The medial septal nucleus and nuclei of the basomedial amygdala project their axons mainly to the medial aspect of the hypothalamus. Raphe neurons, the source of serotonergic fibers that are distributed to all of the forebrain, supply wide regions of the hypothalamus.

488. The answer is B. (Kandel, 3rd Ed., pp. 218, 397-398, 746) When an organism is exposed to stress stimuli, its reaction to other aversive or painful stimuli is suppressed. In fact, the phenomenon of stress-induced analgesia can extend for a considerable period of time (several hours). Stress-induced analgesia is of survival value in that it permits the organism to respond effectively to the stressful stimulus. If the organism responded specifically to the painful stimulus, such a response could be detrimental to its survival, as it might be incompatible with its response to the stressful stimulus. All other choices are correct. Following a stressful event, there is an increase in corticotropin releasing hormone (CRH) from the hypothalamus, which, in turn, results in a release of adrenocorticotrophic hormone (ACTH) from the pituitary. Glucocorticoids, released from the adrenal gland in response to ACTH, inhibit CRH neurons in the hypothalamus. In addition, as a result of stress there is a sudden increase in heart rate and blood pressure. This is most likely due to the activation of descending hypothalamic fibers to lower brainstem nuclei that directly regulate preganglionic sympathetic neurons of the spinal cord. During periods of stress, vasopressin is also released from the supraoptic nucleus. However, the precise mechanism governing the relationship between ACTH and vasopressin release has yet to be elaborated.

489. The answer is C. (Kandel, 3rd Ed., pp. 746-747, 753-756) Stimulation of the medial hypothalamus, especially the ventromedial hypothalamus (and the tissue immediately dorsal), produces a dramatic emotional response in the cat that is referred to as defensive rage behavior. It is characterized by marked sympathetic signs such as increases in heart rate and blood pressure, pupillary dilatation, and piloerection. A behavioral component includes hissing and attempts on the part of the animal to attack another moving animal. One function that is not elicited by stimulation of the medial hypothalamus is feeding. Instead, it can be elicited by stimulation of more lateral regions of hypothalamus.

490. The answer is D. (Kandel, 3rd Ed., p.   756) Lesions of the lateral hypothalamus are likely to produce aphagia. Feeding behavior is elicited by stimulation of the lateral hypothalamus. Neurons in this region respond to the sight or taste of food. Since drinking is also associated with lateral hypothalamic functions, a lesion of this structure would also disrupt this behavior. Lesions of the lateral hypothalamus do not produce either hypertension or sexual behaviors. The neurons regulating these functions are elsewhere within the hypothalamus.

491. The answer is E. (Kandel, 3rd Ed., pp. 752-753) The process of temperature regulation requires the integration of autonomic, skeletomuscular, and endocrine responses. For example, dilation of blood vessels of the skin (an autonomic response) facilitates heat loss while constriction of these vessels helps to conserve heat. Panting and shivering (skeletomuscular responses) aid in the processes of heat loss and conservation (heat generation), respectively. Finally, when an organism is exposed to cold for long periods of time, there is an increase in thyroxine release from the anterior pituitary gland, which helps to increase body temperature by increasing metabolism. The classical interpretation of the role of the hypothalamus in temperature regulation has been that the anterior hypothalamus constitutes a heat loss center, while the posterior hypothalamus is a heat conservation center. Although such a generalization is somewhat oversimplified, the general phenomenon has been demonstrated. For example, stimulation of the anterior hypothalamus has been shown to dilate blood vessels and inhibit shivering and lesions of this region produce hypothermia. Stimulation of the posterior hypothalamus produces heat conservation by constricting blood vessels and causing shivering. Neurons in this region respond to both local warming of hypothalamic tissue as well as to warming of the skin. Neurons in both the septal and preoptic regions constitute antipyretic areas in that they respond to increases in fever by limiting the magnitude of the fever. Activation of these antipyretic regions is thought to occur through a mechanism utilizing the peptide vasopressin. The precise mechanism by which these regions become activated remains unknown.

492. The answer is D. (Kandel, 3rd Ed., pp. 758, 801-802) Recent studies have demonstrated that the suprachiasmatic nucleus controls the biological clock of internal circadian rhythms. During the light phase of the light-dark cycle, metabolic activity (measured by ^{14}C-2-deoxyglucose autoradiography) within the suprachiasmatic nucleus is significantly increased. In contrast, during the dark phase, there is very little metabolic activity present.

493. The answer is B. (Carpenter and Sutin, 8th Ed., pp. 634-636) The amygdala and prefrontal cortex share reciprocal connections, but their functional nature has not been clearly resolved. The amygdala receives inputs from the hypothalamus which might provide the anatomical basis for a feedback relationship between the two sets of structures. Inputs from the locus ceruleus involve norepinephrine fibers. The most prominent sensory inputs involve olfaction which come from mitral cell axons passing from the olfactory bulb to the corticomedial amygdala. The cingulate gyrus does not project to the amygdala. Instead, its limbic projections are directed mainly to the hippocampal formation.

494. The answer is C. (Carpenter and Sutin, 8th Ed., p. 636) One of the most interesting discoveries concerning the amygdala made in recent years is that the central nucleus contains high concentrations of a number of peptides. These include enkephalins and somatostatin in particular. This region also receives large numbers of dopaminergic axon terminals as well. The central nucleus does not project its axons to the medial hypothalamus. It does not receive auditory or visual signals, nor does it project to the spinal cord where it could inhibit spinal motor neurons. It receives norepinephrine-containing fibers from the brainstem rather than being a source of this neurotransmitter.

495. The answer is B. (Kandel, 3rd Ed., p. 747) In this syndrome, produced experimentally in monkeys and also seen in cats, there is an extreme change in the personality of the animal. Its responses to emotional-laden stimuli are much reduced. It appears very tame. Aggressive tendencies are not evident. It also manifests oral tendencies and displays hypersexuality. This syndrome is the result of lesions of the temporal lobe in which parts of the amygdala are involved. Lesions of other regions such as the hypothalamus, cingulate cortex, or septal area do not produce the Kluver-Bucy syndrome.

496. The answer is D. (Carpenter and Sutin, 8th Ed., pp. 632-634) Extensive research on the hippocampal formation has revealed that it is involved in a wide variety of functions. The hippocampal formation plays a role in the control of emotional behavior. Tumors of this structure have resulted in marked changes in emotional aspects of personality such as the expression of intense anger to a normally innocuous situation. In addition, since this region has a very low threshold for the onset of seizure activity, tumors of the hippocampus most frequently result in the development of seizures such as psychomotor epilepsy. A unique feature of the hippocampus is its association with short-term memory (recent memory) functions. For example, damage to this structure makes it very difficult for individuals to remember information to which they have just been exposed (although they may easily remember many events in their distant past). Because of the relationship of the hippocampal formation to the hypothalamus directly via the fornix or indirectly via the septal region, tumors of the hippocampal formation may lead to significant changes in endocrine function. However, there is no evidence to suggest that the hippocampal formation plays a role in temperature regulation. This function is known to be more closely associated with the anterior hypothalamus, preoptic region, and possibly neighboring parts of the septal area.

497. The answer is D. (Carpenter and Sutin, 8th Ed., p. 631) A major target of efferent fibers from the hippocampal formation is the septal area. Fibers located in the precommissural fornix supply the septal area in an extensive and topographical manner. In turn, the septal area projects significant numbers of fibers to the lateral (and medial) regions of hypothalamus. In this manner, the septal area serves as a relay for the transmission of signals from the hippocampal formation to the hypothalamus. The hippocampal formation does not project to the habenular nuclei, mediodorsal nucleus, or the bed nucleus of stria terminalis. Moreover, the cingulate gyrus does not project directly to the hypothalamus.

498. The answer is C. (Noback and Demarest, 3rd Ed., pp. 474-475; Carpenter and Sutin, 8th Ed., pp. 632-633) For many years, it was believed that a neural circuit composed of the hippocampal formation —> mammillary bodies —> anterior thalamic nucleus —> cingulate gyrus —> hippocampal formation played a major role in the regulation of emotional behavior. More recent studies by a number of investigators have revealed that neither the mammillary bodies nor anterior thalamic nucleus appears to contribute to the regulation of emotional behavior. Instead, it is believed that this circuit may subserve functions more closely related to short-term memory.

499. The answer is B. (Carpenter and Sutin, 8th Ed., pp. 544, 644-705) The cerebrovascular accident produced damage of the right primary visual cortex. Therefore, this would result in a homonymous hemianopsia of the left visual fields. Since the damage was confined to the occipital lobe, there would be little effect upon other processes such as speech, motor functions, or intellectual activities.

500. The answer is C. (Carpenter and Sutin, 8th Ed., pp. 714-721) The occipital lobe is supplied by the posterior cerebral artery. The calcarine cortex (primary visual cortex) is supplied by a branch of this artery which is called the calcarine artery. The anterior cerebral artery supplies the medial aspect of the frontal lobe and the anterior-medial aspect of the parietal lobe. The middle cerebral artery supplies the lateral aspect of the frontal and parietal lobes. The superior cerebellar artery supplies the dorsolateral aspect of a portion of the pons and the cerebellum. The striate arteries arise from the anterior and middle cerebral arteries and supply portions of the internal capsule and neostriatum.

501. The answer is A. (Carpenter and Sutin, 8th Ed., p. 583, see Fig. 17-5) The tumor is situated in the lentiform nucleus and internal capsule. Therefore, corticospinal fibers will be affected, causing an upper motor neuron paralysis of the left side. Dyskinesia would not be seen because any effects normally seen in association with damage to the basal ganglia would be masked by the effects of the damage to the internal capsule. Since the cerebellum was not involved, there would be no intention tremor. Neither would there be any visual deficits from this glioma since optic nerve fibers are not involved. The schematic diagram below indicates the approximate extent of the tumor. Labeled are the caudate nucleus (C), globus pallidus (GP), the internal capsule (IC), the putamen (P), and the tumor (T).

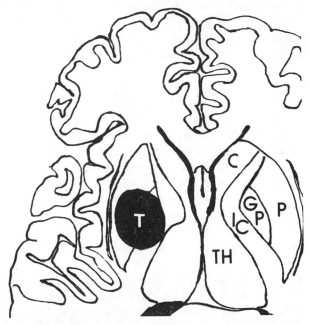

502. The answer is D. (Carpenter and Sutin, 8th Ed., p.583, Fig. 17-5) The tumor clearly involves the lentiform nucleus of the basal ganglia and has expanded to include the internal capsule as well. At the stage when the CT scan was taken, the tumor had not involved the thalamus.

503. The answer is B. (Carpenter and Sutin, 8th Ed., pp. 704-705) The tumor involves the prefrontal cortex. This region of the cortex is associated with a number of important functions that would be affected by the tumor. Damage to the prefrontal cortex typically results in intellectual deficits such as a loss of problem-solving ability and response perseveration. It also produces significant effects upon emotional behavior, such as a flat affect. In addition, seizures are a natural consequence of the presence of tumors, which have an irritating effect upon nerve cells. Paralysis would not occur because the tumor did not damage the primary or secondary motor cortices.

504. The answer is E. (Carpenter and Sutin; 8th Ed., pp. 694-697) The prefrontal cortex maintains reciprocal connections with both the mediodorsal thalamic nucleus and amygdala. In addition, the prefrontal cortex supplies the basilar pons (fronto-pontine fibers) and contributes fibers (as part of the overall projection from the frontal lobe) to the neostriatum. The prefrontal cortex, however, does not project to the lateral geniculate nucleus of the thalamus.

505. The answer is C. (Carpenter and Sutin, 8th Ed., pp. 684-695, 702-704) The arterial occlusion involves both the temporal and occipital regions of cortex. Therefore, it would affect Wernicke's area as well as primary visual areas of the occipital lobe. Thus, the patient would most likely present with receptive aphasia as well as a right homonymous hemianopsia. It would not likely produce marked intellectual deficits since the prefrontal cortex was spared; nor would it produce hemiballism since there was no damage to the subthalamic nucleus.

506. The answer is B. (Carpenter and Sutin, 8th Ed., pp. 717-718) Although the tissue affected involves parietal, temporal, and occipital lobes, the primary artery affected is the middle cerebral artery. The unusual feature about this occlusion is that it appears that the middle cerebral artery extends more caudally than usual. Nevertheless, the middle cerebral artery is the only one (of the choices presented) that could account for the damage to the temporal and parietal cortices. The anterior cerebral artery supplies the medial aspects of the frontal and parietal lobes; the posterior cerebral artery supplies the occipital cortex (visual areas); the posterior choroidal artery mainly supplies part of the tectum, medial and superior aspects of the thalamus, and the choroid plexus of the third ventricle. The superior cerebellar artery supplies the dorsolateral aspect of a portion of the pons and cerebellum.

507. The answer is B. (Carpenter and Sutin, 8th Ed., pp. 718-721) An arterial occlusion compromised the blood supply to the occipital lobe on the left side of the brain. Therefore, it would result in a right homonymous hemianopsia with no motor deficits (since no motor regions of the brain are affected).

508. The answer is E. (Carpenter and Sutin, 8th Ed., pp. 718-721) This vertebral angiogram is an anterior view of the back of the brain. It reveals an occlusion of the left posterior cerebral artery (A). It should be noted that the posterior cerebral arteries are formed from the bifurcation of the basilar artery. Follow the basilar artery caudally (see bottom of the photograph) to the position where it is connected to the vertebral arteries.

509. The answer is D. (Carpenter and Sutin, 8th Ed., p. 544) This large pituitary tumor is seen to compress the optic chiasm. Damage to the chiasm affects the crossing fibers of the nasal retina which convey information from the temporal visual fields. This results in a bitemporal hemianopsia. Since some parts of the optic nerves are spared, pupillary reflexes are preserved. The neuroanatomical substrates for conjugate gaze (i.e., frontal eye fields, pontine gaze center, medial longitudinal fasciculus (MLF), and nuclei of cranial nerves III, IV, and VI) are unaffected by the tumor; the mechanism of conjugate gaze remains intact.

Bibliography

Carpenter, M.B., Sutin, J. *Human Neuroanatomy*, 8th Ed., Baltimore, Williams and Wilkins, 1983.

Cooper, J.R., Bloom, F.E., Roth, R.H., *The Biochemical Basis of Neuropharmacology*, 6th Ed., New York, Oxford University Press, 1991.

DeArmond, S.J., Fusco, M.M., Dewey, M.M., *Structure of the Human Brain*, 3rd Ed., New York, Oxford University Press, 1989.

Guyton, A.C., *Basic Neuroscience*, 2nd Ed., Philadelphia, W.B. Saunders, 1991.

Kandel, E.R., Schwartz, J.H., Jessel, T.M., *Principles of Neural Science*, 3rd Ed., New York, Elsevier, 1991.

Villiger, E., Ludwig, E., Rasmussen, A.T., *Atlas of Cross Section Anatomy of the Brain*, New York, McGraw-Hill, 1951.

Wilson, J.D., et al, *Harrison's Principle's of Internal Medicine*, 12th Ed., New York, McGraw-Hill, 1991.

Wilson-Pauwels, L., Akesson, E.J., Stewart, P.A., *Cranial Nerves*, Toronto, B.C. Decker Inc., 1988.